Fast Tract Digestion
Heartburn

Norman Robillard, Ph.D.

Founder, Digestive Health Institute

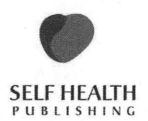

SELF HEALTH
PUBLISHING

Self Health Publishing

Watertown, Massachusetts

First edition
ISBN 978-0-9766425-3-4

Recipes: Rie Tanaka

Editor: Edward Walters

Figures: Mahesh Gudapakkam

Cover design: Karrie Ross

Disclaimers

Acknowledgements

The research and writing of this book was supported by the efforts of several people.

Rie Tanaka was the creative force behind the recipes in the book. Her innate knowledge and creativity in the preparation and presentation of American and Japanese cuisine give the recipes in this book their special appeal, winning the praise of those enrolled in the clinical study of the Fast Tract Diet.

Gary Taubes helped me gain perspective on the limitations of observational studies particularly with regard to the health aspects of fiber.

Dr. Mike Eades was supportive of my research asking key questions that helped me focus on the real problem.

My editor, Ed Walters, made sure the ideas in the book were organized and simplified to help the reader cut to the chase and gain the maximum benefit from the information.

Mahesh Gudapakkam, re-created the figures in this book to improve their resolution for printing.

Karrie Ross designed the book cover in a way that highlights the books value and conveys the importance of this new approach in treating acid reflux.

Table of Contents

Table of Contents

Introduction

Almost fifteen years ago, Elaine Gottschall, in her book, *Breaking the Vicious Cycle*, proposed that faulty digestion could lead to the malabsorption of certain sugars, starches and fibers and ultimately result in the overgrowth of bacteria in the small intestine. These overgrowing bacteria can cause injury to the lining of the small intestine thus impairing digestion and causing even more malabsorption. She linked this cycle of overgrowth, injury and malabsorption with several digestive conditions including irritable bowel syndrome, Crohn's disease, ulcerative colitis, diverticulitis, celiac disease, and chronic diarrhea.

Fast Tract Digestion — Heartburn, the first in a series of books on digestive illness, picks up where *Breaking the Vicious Cycle* left off. My research on the root cause of acid reflux can be summed up in two conclusions:

> *(1) Acid reflux is linked to cycles of carbohydrate malabsorption and bacterial overgrowth in the small intestine. The overgrowing bacteria produce intestinal gas which drives acid reflux — much like dropping a Mentos in a bottle of Coke.*

> *(2) Limiting your consumption of five specific types of difficult-to-digest carbohydrates can help you prevent this bacterial overgrowth and provide an effective treatment for this condition.*

Fast Tract Digestion explains the connection between digestion, malabsorption, bacteria and chronic acid reflux.

I describe the three basic food groups and how optimal digestion and absorption supports digestive health. Then I explore the various scenarios that can lead to malabsorption and bacterial overgrowth, which can result in the dramatic symptoms of chronic acid reflux. The biggest problem — difficult to digest carbohydrates driving bacterial overgrowth — is examined in depth.

Finally, *Fast Tract Digestion* provides a new type of clinically proven dietary treatment plan for people suffering from the wide variety of symptoms resulting from chronic acid reflux.

Chapter 1: What is GERD?

Approximately sixty million people in the US report that they suffer at least once a week from the symptoms of acid reflux, making it one of the most common, and most debilitating, digestive conditions that many people will ever face.[1]

GERD, which stands for GastroEsophageal Reflux Disease, is a chronic condition caused by the repeated refluxing of stomach contents into the esophagus. In other words, GERD and chronic acid reflux is the same thing.

The most common symptom is heartburn, which most people with GERD describe as a burning sensation behind their breastbone. Other symptoms of GERD can include abdominal pain, coughing, a sour taste in their mouth, sore throat, hoarseness, laryngitis, asthma-like symptoms, and sinus irritation. Smoking, pregnancy, obesity, hiatal hernia (where the stomach protrudes into the esophagus through a tear or weakness of the diaphragm that separates them) and even tight-fitting clothes can make these symptoms worse.

How is GERD Diagnosed?

Diagnosing GERD is relatively straight forward, even though successful long-term treatment or a cure for this condition has proven elusive for mainstream medical science.

Most people are diagnosed with GERD after their doctor has reviewed their history of symptoms in detail, including the frequency of their heartburn, or the related symptoms described above. This information is more than enough to lead most doctors to prescribe over-the-counter medicines, or proton pump inhibitor (PPI) medicines for more severe cases.

Both types of medicines are designed to significantly reduce the amount of acid in your stomach. If your symptoms improve as a result of treatment, your doctor will probably conclude that you have GERD. If further diagnostic tests are necessary, the doctor may also recommend upper gastrointestinal endoscopy. One of the best indicators of GERD is damage or irritation to the lining of the esophagus. Endoscopy lets your doctor look at the lining of your esophagus, stomach, and the first part of your small intestine through a miniature camera.

Additional tests can include manometry, a procedure that measures how tightly your lower esophageal sphincter (also known as your LES, this is the "valve" that separates your stomach and your esophagus) closes, along with 24 hour pH monitoring which detects how much acid is leaking into your esophagus, and how long it remains there.

How is GERD Treated?

The leading contemporary theory for the cause of GERD suggests that certain (trigger) foods, for example caffeine, or alcohol, can relax or weaken the LES muscles, making it possible for stomach acid to "leak" into your esophagus, causing the typical burning sensation.

Today's standard treatments for GERD fall into three basic categories: acid-reducing medications, surgery, and dietary changes.

Medications

Medications in order of increasing potency include:

> *Over-the-counter antacids, such as* Tums, Rolaids, Gaviscon *and* Maalox, *which chemically neutralize stomach acids;*
>
> *Histamine antagonists (H2 antagonists) such as famotidine* (Pepcid), *cimetidine* (Tagamet), *nizatidine* (Axid), *and ranitadine* (Zantac), *which are used for milder reflux symptoms, and usually available over-the-counter; and*
>
> *Prescription-strength Proton Pump Inhibitors (PPIs) such as esomeprazole* (Nexium), *omeprazole* (Prilosec *and* Zegerid), *lansoprazole* (Prevacid), *pantoprazole* (Protonix) *and rabeprazole* (Aciphex). *PPIs are prescribed for more severe GERD symptoms. A few PPI drugs,* Prilosec OTC *and* Zegerid OTC, *for example, are also now available over-the-counter.*

Antacids neutralize stomach acid while H2 antagonists and PPI drugs block the production of acid by specialized parietal cells that line the stomach. All of these medications are applied regularly in the treatment of GERD, but they also create a number of new issues:

Acid-reducing drugs, malabsorption and bacteria. Acid-reducing drugs can significantly reduce the level of acid in your stomach. The hope is that if your stomach contents "reflux" or escape into your esophagus, these reduced acid levels will also reduce the burning sensation and tissue damage caused by the acid. While this approach does control some GERD symptoms, acid-reducing drugs do not control bloating, belching, gas, and regurgitation.

PPIs have also been linked to significant side effects and long-term health risks.

Because these drugs neutralize stomach acid, the absorption of vitamins, minerals and nutrients can be negatively affected and bacteria are more able to colonize the stomach and overgrow in the small intestine making the underlying problem worse and affecting the levels of bile acids needed for fat digestion.[2]

Acid-suppressing drugs and C diff. C diff (Clostridium difficile) is a dangerous gut pathogen, and *C diff* infections can cause symptoms ranging from severe diarrhea to life-threatening inflammation of the colon. Recently, *C diff* infections have become more frequent, more severe, and much more difficult to treat.

One cause of this development is the overuse of broad-spectrum antibiotics, which wipe out friendly bacteria, but these infections have also been linked to both PPI drugs and H2 blockers.[3]

Even more troubling, PPI drugs lower the *C diff* cure rate and increase the rate of reinfection.[4]

Acid suppressing drugs and pneumonia. We will discuss the causes and treatment of bacterial overgrowth at great length later in this book. At this point it's only important to know that Small Intestinal Bacterial Overgrowth (or SIBO) can actually spread beyond the digestive tract. Normally, stomach acid kills bacteria, so that intestinal bacteria can't reach your esophagus, lungs, and sinuses. However, when acid-reducing drugs (PPIs, H2 blockers and even antacids) are used, bacteria from the intestines can survive in the stomach.

Once in your stomach or upper small intestine, the bacteria can reach your esophagus, and potentially your lungs and sinuses, through "reflux" of your stomach's contents past your LES.

It's been proven that people taking acid-blocking medications are more susceptible to respiratory infections from bacteria likely originating in their own intestines. A study of more than 364,000 people, led by Robert J.F. Laheij at the University Medical Center at St. Radboud in Nijmegen, the Netherlands, found that the risk of pneumonia almost doubled in people taking proton-pump inhibitors for prolonged periods of time.[5] This increased risk of respiratory infection was also seen in a second study of children taking acid-reducing medications.[6]

3

PPI drugs and bone fractures. According to a study in the Journal of the American Medical Association (JAMA), the long term use of PPIs can lead to weakened bones and more frequent fractures.[7] When researchers compared 13,556 subjects with previous hip fractures with 13,386 control subjects, they found that the subjects who had taken PPIs for as little as one year had a 44 percent higher risk of breaking a hip. Even more troubling, subjects taking PPIs in high doses for long periods of time increased their risk of hip fracture by 245 percent.

Calcium is absorbed efficiently only when the stomach is acidic. The authors of this study suggested that the increased risk of fracture might be due to PPIs interfering with calcium metabolism.

In fact, the increased risk of fracture includes not only the hip, but the wrist and spine, as well. The FDA reviewed several epidemiological studies of people over 50 years old taking PPI drugs, and reported that the greatest risk was for those taking high doses of PPI drugs for more than one year. Subsequently, the FDA has required changes to product labels to disclose the additional risks.

PPI drugs and low magnesium levels. In March 2011, the FDA informed the public (information on FDA.gov web site) that taking prescription PPI drugs or for extended periods (over one year in most cases) could cause low serum magnesium levels (hypomagnesemia) consistent with low intestinal absorption of magnesium. This deficiency in magnesium blood levels (similar in some way to calcium deficiency) can result in a number of serious symptoms including muscle cramps, involuntary movements, cardiac arrhythmia, hypertension, and central nervous system problems including irritability, confusion, hallucinations, depression and seizures. The FDA went on to say that dietary supplementation of magnesium did not correct the problem in about 25% of the cases and PPI drugs needed to be discontinued.

The warning was not extended to over-the-counter PPIs because these drugs are marketed at lower doses and indicated for shorter treatment durations (14 days three times per year). However, taking higher doses or taking OTC PPIs long term would certainly present the same risk.

Surgery

Surgery is a more radical and invasive approach to controlling acid reflux. One procedure, known as Nissen Fundoplication, seeks to improve the barrier between the esophagus and stomach by strengthening the lower

4

esophageal sphincter. The surgeon pulls up the very top part of the stomach and tightly secures it around the esophagus with sutures effectively tightening the LES.

Though this procedure has been moderately successful at controlling reflux, a significant number of patients report a range of new symptoms following the surgery.

These can include breakthrough reflux, excessive gas, flatulence, abdominal bloating, inability to vomit or belch, diarrhea, stomach pain and difficulty swallowing. People experiencing these side effects may require PPI drug therapy after the operation, or even multiple procedures.

As with the medications we looked at above, fundoplication does not treat the underlying condition, but in this case focuses on containing the stomach acid that causes the symptoms.

Dietary Changes

The standard dietary advice for people suffering from GERD is based on the idea that a link exists between the foods you eat and acid reflux. This "trigger food" approach recommends eliminating specific foods that cause reflux from your diet.

There are a number of problems with this approach. First, it seems impossible to identify cause and effect between specific foods and symptoms. You can get heartburn from something you ate one hour ago, or six hours ago. That means that it's easy to misidentify which food really caused your symptoms.

Another problem is that most meals combine different foods that belong to all three major food groups (proteins, fats and carbohydrates), and it's difficult to assign blame to any one ingredient. For example, it's easy to blame your heartburn on the spicy tomato sauce on your pizza, even though the real problem was the high-amylose wheat flour in the crust.

A number of foods have been implicated as potential "triggers" for acid reflux. Trigger foods reportedly include fried foods, citrus fruits, dairy products, tomatoes and other acidic foods, fats and oils, spices, beverages like coffee, wine, beer and soft drinks, and sweets like cookies and chocolate. By the way, fats and oils have been implicated based only on their association with fried foods that are often breaded or batter dipped with flour high in resistant starch. Evidence exists in the scientific literature that fats do not cause reflux [8,9].

You may rightly wonder, "Why would so many different types of foods trigger acid reflux? And what is left for me to eat?" A common thread that explains how and why trigger foods cause symptoms has proved elusive. In general, diets that limit trigger foods have been ineffective — resulting in soaring sales of acid-reducing medicines.

The Fast Tract Approach to GERD

I'm going to suggest that there's a different way of looking at GERD, one that accounts for the latest developments in medical science, and one that proposes a radically different way of treating GERD.

I believe that GERD is not caused by mysterious trigger foods or other substances that "relax" the LES muscles, but rather by gases produced by the common bacteria we harbor in our intestines.

This gas can create higher pressure in the small intestine and stomach, and ultimately power acid reflux. People with weakened or damaged LES muscles will be even more susceptible to reflux, because it will take less gas pressure to propel the stomach contents past the LES.

This idea came as a surprise to many people when I first wrote about it in my book, *Heartburn Cured*.[10]

But the Fast Tract Diet is based on good research and the latest developments in medical science. The Fast Tract approach, based on limiting foods that are difficult to digest, and reducing the overgrowth of bacteria in the small intestine, is the first to identify the cause-and-effect relationship between known biological processes and GERD.

It's also the first to offer a sound, safe, practical program for managing your diet so that you can eliminate your symptoms altogether, or at least reduce them to an absolute minimum.

A Clinically Proven Diet

My initial research suggested that the Fast Tract Diet should be effective at controlling all of the symptoms of chronic acid reflux. As a long time heartburn sufferer, I used the diet to treat my own chronic reflux with complete success, but would the diet work on other people with this condition?

To test the diet, I teamed up with a clinical researcher with experience in GERD studies and put together a clinical study to evaluate the effectiveness of this diet in 19 people from the Boston area who suffered from chronic acid reflux symptoms at least three times per week.

Initially, participants were instructed to consume their normal diet for 7 days (period 1) while recording their symptoms.

Next, participants were placed on the Fast Tract Diet for 7 days (period 2) and instructed to continue recording their symptoms. The results were nothing short of amazing. As indicated in the graph below, all acid reflux related symptoms measured decreased dramatically after being on the diet for only one week!

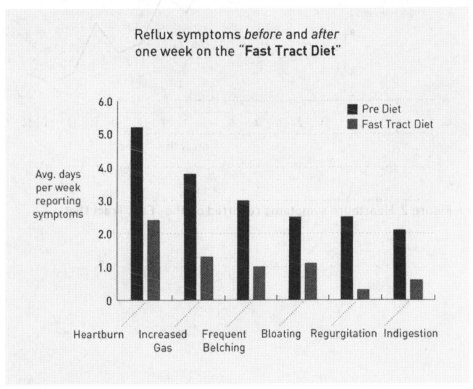

Figure 1. Summary results for the "Fast Tract Diet"

What's even more impressive is the decrease over time of all GERD-related symptoms. The following graphs show the actual results on a day by day basis for each of the reflux-related symptoms.

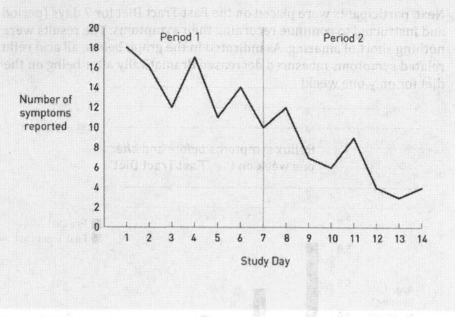
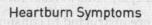

Figure 2. Heartburn symptoms reported on the "**Fast Tract Diet**"

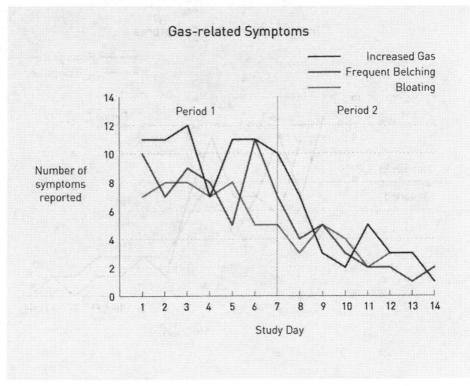

Figure 3. Gas-related symptoms reported on the "**Fast Tract Diet**"

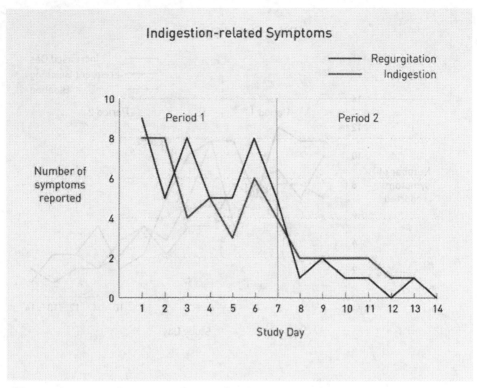

Figure 4. Indigestion-related symptoms reported on the "**Fast Tract Diet**"

By the end of one week on the diet, most subjects reported no symptoms at all! The progressive improvement of all GERD-related symptoms over time is evidence for the effectiveness of the Fast Tract Diet. Most of the reported symptoms occur during the first part of the week. While continued study on this approach is warranted, the results from this clinical study clearly support the concept behind the Fast Tract Diet approach.

Chapter 2: Food Chemistry

The purpose of the next two chapters is to provide a basic framework on what food is made of, how each food type is digested, and how our body uses food. Reading this chapter will make the concept of malabsorption and bacterial overgrowth easier to understand.

The Fast Tract Diet that I'm introducing here is based on medical science and biological chemistry. I know it works because I've researched this approach fully, used it in treating my own GERD symptoms, and tested the diet in a controlled clinical study. But unless you're a doctor or nutritionist by trade, you may not understand why the Fast Tract program is such a breakthrough in treating GERD, or why it's so important that you follow the program carefully to get the results you want.

The basic connection you need to understand is between the digestion and absorption (or, really, the incomplete digestion and malabsorption) of food, how it leads to Small Intestinal Bacterial Overgrowth (SIBO) and, in turn, to GastroEsophageal Reflux Disorder (GERD). In order to understand how they're linked in your body, and why my approach to treating them is plausible, you need to know a little more about the basics of human digestion.

In this chapter I'm going to introduce the three basic types of food — what they're made of and how they are digested.

The Three Basic Types of Food

Given the tremendous variety of foods available, it may seem surprising that all foods fall into only three categories: carbohydrates, proteins, and fats. Fats and carbohydrates satisfy most of our energy needs, but we need protein to grow, repair damaged cells and make new proteins including critical enzymes, antibodies and structural molecules.

Animal-based foods like beef, pork, poultry, fish, dairy products, and eggs are rich in both proteins and fats. Vegetables, fruits and grains are rich sources of carbohydrates. However, many plant-based foods are also good sources of proteins and fats. Animal-based foods contain negligible amounts of carbohydrates.

Carbohydrates

The primary role of the carbohydrates in our diet is to help us meet our need for energy. Plant-based foods such as fruits, vegetables, grains, pasta, flours, potatoes, pastries, candy, rice, sugar and breads contain mostly carbohydrates. Carbohydrates include sugars, starches and fibers and are made up of the elements carbon, hydrogen and oxygen. Glucose, a sugar, is the carbohydrate our cells like to use to get energy. Most of the carbohydrates we eat are eventually broken down to glucose, and burned by our cells for fuel, or stored as glycogen or fat. (A quick note here: carbohydrates are also the preferred food of bacteria. More on this later.)

Monosaccharides

The basic carbohydrate unit is called a monosaccharide, meaning "single sugar." Single sugars do not really require digestion; they can be absorbed directly from the intestine into your blood. Monosaccharides include sugars like glucose, fructose and galactose. Glucose is the most common and important monosaccharide — it is your body's basic food.

Monosaccharides can link together to form more complex carbohydrates that do require digestion. For example, disaccharides (made up of two sugar units) such as lactose and sucrose, or polysaccharides (made up of multiple sugar units) such as raffinose (made up of three sugars), stachyose (made up of four sugars), or starches and fiber (made up of thousands to millions of sugar units).

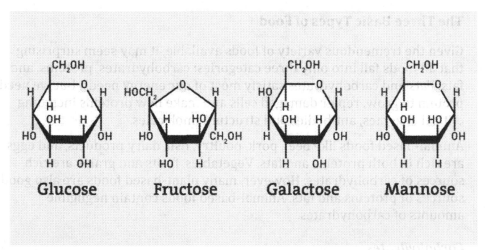

Glucose   Fructose   Galactose   Mannose

Figure 5. Monosaccharides

Disaccharides

Disaccharides are composed of two sugars and must be broken down into monosaccharides to be absorbed into the blood stream. Disaccharides include sucrose, made up of glucose and fructose, and commonly known as table sugar; lactose, made up of glucose and galactose, and commonly known as milk sugar; and maltose, produced by the breakdown of starch, and made up of two glucose molecules.

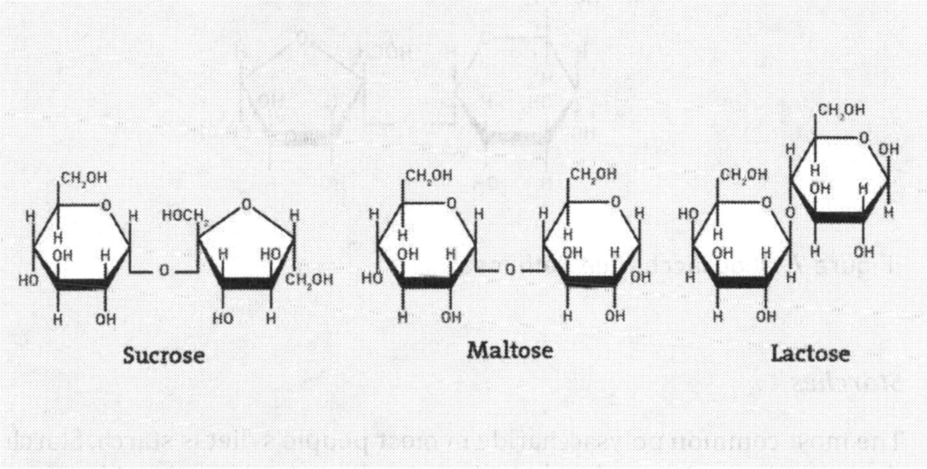

Sucrose   Maltose   Lactose

Figure 6. Disaccharides

Polysaccharides

Polysaccharides are made up of multiple sugar units. Smaller sugar chains called oligosaccharides include stachyose and raffinose. Starches, including amylose and amylopectin, and fibers including cellulose, hemicellulose and pectin are composed of thousands to millions of repeating glucose units. Both of these types of polysaccharides will play extremely important roles in the following chapters.
Oligosaccharides

Oligosaccharides are short polysaccharides containing between three and ten sugar units. Examples include fructose oligosaccharide (FOS), made from repeating fructose units and found in many plants; stachyose, composed of glucose, fructose, and two galactose sugar units and found in beans and vegetables; and raffinose, composed of glucose, fructose and galactose. Because these oligosaccharides are non- or only marginally digestible, they are defined as dietary fiber.

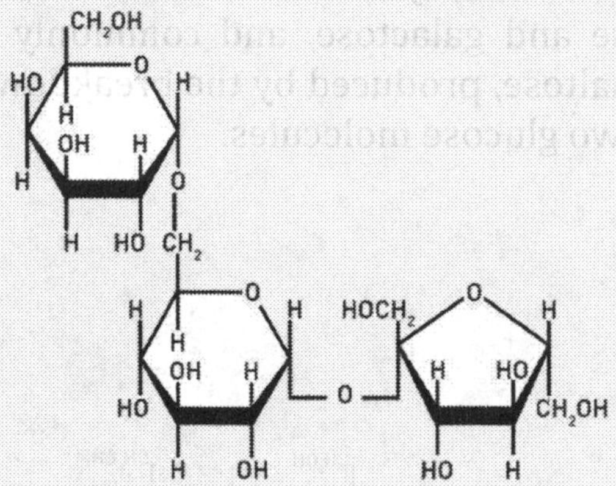

Figure 7. Oligosaccharide Raffinose

Starches

The most common polysaccharide in most people's diet is starch. Starch is the major form of stored carbohydrate in plants, and is present in grain foods like wheat, rice, corn, oats and barley as well as tubers like potatoes.

Most starchy plants contain two types of starch, amylose, an essentially linear polysaccharide, and amylopectin, a more complex and highly branched polysaccharide. Both are composed entirely of glucose sugar units. Most starchy vegetables (including corn, wheat, oats and most barley, as well as many varieties of rice and potatoes) contain 20 to 30% amylose and 70 to 80% amylopectin. Some potatoes, corn and legumes contain higher percentages (up to 65 percent or more) of amylose. Some plant varieties like waxy rice (also known as short grain, glutinous, sweet or sticky rice) and waxy barley may contain up to 100% amylopectin. This is important for our discussion because one of these starch types, amylose, is very difficult to digest.

Amylopectin

Amylopectin can contain up to 2 million glucose units. Its structure is more complex than amylose with branches up to 30 glucose units long occurring every 25 to 30 glucose units or so. Due to amylopectin's branching and less dense structure, amylopectin is much easier to break down to glucose than amylose. The main enzyme responsible for the breakdown of amylopectin is amylase, which is found both in our saliva and our small intestine.

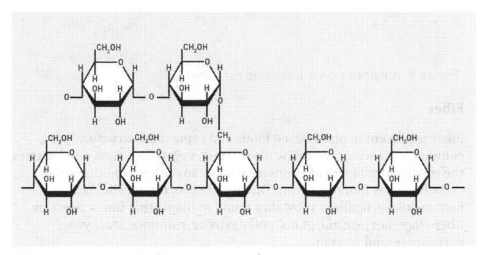

Figure 8. Amylopectin *(branching shown)*

Amylose

Amylose starch molecules are much smaller than amylopectin, containing as few as several hundred to as many as several thousand glucose molecules. Amylose is also broken down by the enzyme amylase, but less efficiently than amylopectin, because the amylose molecule has fewer branch points and can be packed more tightly into starch granules.

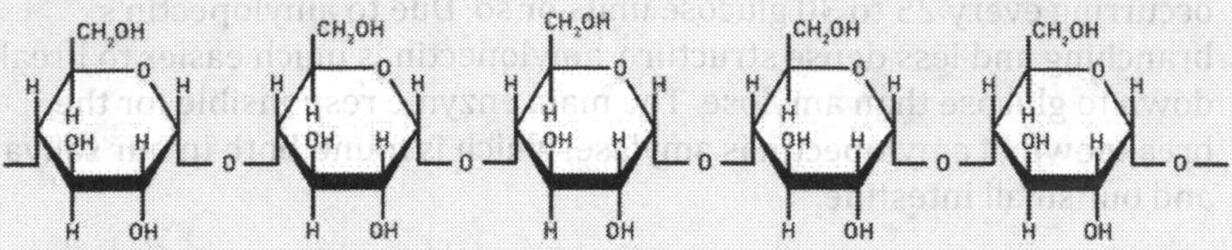

Figure 9. Amylose *(minor branching not shown)*

Fiber

Fiber is present in plant-based foods and represents structural components such as the cell walls of fruits, vegetables, nuts and legumes, the tough outer layers of grains, as well as any other non- digestible carbohydrates found in plants. Dietary fiber includes cellulose, hemicellulose, lignin (a substance found in plants that binds cellulose fibers together), pectin, gums, polydextrose, raffinose, stachyose, verbascose, and fructans.

Resistant starch is sometimes also considered a class of dietary fiber. But unlike starch, fiber is not digestible by humans. We lack the enzymes to break the chemical bonds between the sugar molecules in fiber. The molecular structure of one type of fiber, cellulose, is shown below.

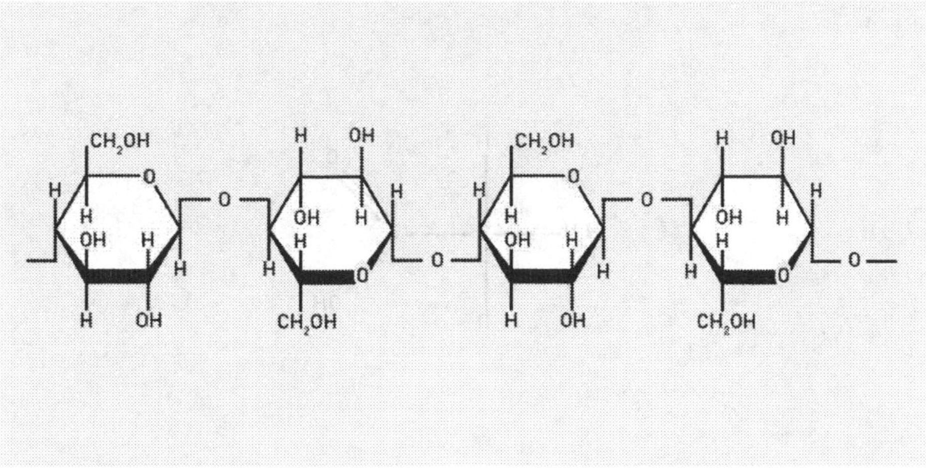

Figure 10. Cellulose

Proteins

Foods such as meats, poultry, fish, eggs and cheese are mostly protein but also contain fats. Protein can also be found in foods such as nuts, beans, grains and seeds. Proteins are generally large molecules that are composed of specific building blocks known as amino acids (see figure 11). As with carbohydrates, proteins contain the elements carbon, hydrogen and oxygen, but proteins also contain nitrogen and sulfur.

Proteins can be used for energy or to make new proteins. Amino acids are required for muscle growth, the repair of damaged cells, and to make enzymes, hormones and structural proteins such as collagen. Approximately half of all amino acids can be made by our body and are known as "non-essential" amino acids. Our bodies cannot produce the other amino acid, and they must be supplied in our diet — or by the microorganisms living in our intestinal tract. These are referred to as "essential" amino acids.

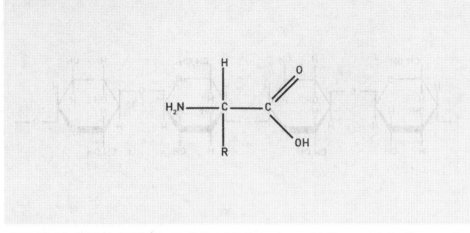

Figure 11. Amino Acid *(the building block amino acids have unique R groups. Glycine's R group is a single hydrogen (H) atom, while Alanine's R group is a methyl (CH3) group)*

To make new proteins, amino acids are linked together via peptide bonds. The peptide bonds form the backbone of the protein, which can be thought of as a long chain. Twenty different amino acids are used to compose proteins. Proteins range in size from about 40 amino acids (smaller proteins are referred to as peptides) to hundreds of amino acids. The sequence of the amino acids in the protein chain determine its primary structure but proteins can fold back onto themselves in such a way as to have secondary and tertiary structures. The shape of a "re-folded" protein is held in place by a weak force called hydrogen bonding. Proteins are much more complex than carbohydrates or fats because of these secondary and tertiary structures, but their complex shapes make their many catalytic, regulatory, and structural applications possible.

A quick side note about proteins: Proteins that are not digested and fully absorbed can be selectively metabolized by intestinal bacteria but are less likely to contribute to SIBO and intestinal gas.

Fats

Fats have gotten a bad name in the diet business. In fact, fats comprise a significant part of a normal diet, and you need to eat an adequate amount of healthy fats to maintain your health. Fats provide both an excellent energy source, as well as building materials for cell membranes, hormones and other fatty acid-based molecules.

Good dietary sources of fats include meat, poultry, fish, eggs, cheese, butter, vegetable oils, nuts, and avocados. Fats are also found in smaller amounts in grains and green leafy vegetables.

Like carbohydrates, fats are comprised of the elements hydrogen, oxygen and carbon. Fatty acids are the "building blocks" of fats. (Just as amino acids are the building blocks of proteins, and sugars are the building blocks of carbohydrates).

Chemically, all fats have the same -COOH (carboxylic acid) group at the end of carbon chains ranging from 4 to 29 carbons in length.

There are four different kinds of fats: mono-unsaturated fats, poly-unsaturated fats, saturated fats and hydrogenated or trans-fats. These categories are based on the bonding structures within the carbon chains.

Monounsaturated fats are found in nuts, peanut oil, olive oil, canola oil, meats and butter, while polyunsaturated fats (refer to figure 12), are found in fish as well as canola, safflower and flaxseed oil. Both monounsaturated and polyunsaturated fats are believed to have significant health benefits because they lower bad cholesterol (LDL) and increase good cholesterol (HDL).

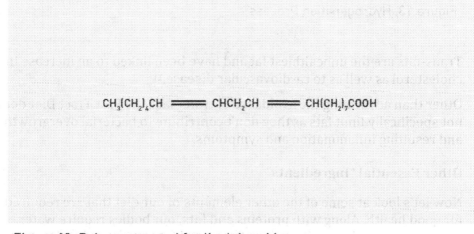

$$CH_3(CH_2)_4CH = CHCH_2CH = CH(CH_2)_7COOH$$

Figure 12. Polyunsaturated fat linoleic acid

Saturated fats are found in many foods including butter, cream, coconut oil, palm oil, poultry and meats. They have been associated with an increase in both good (HDL) and bad (LDL) cholesterol. There is a growing consensus that a certain amount of saturated fats may actually be healthy for our bodies, especially our immune systems, and should be consumed along with mono- and polyunsaturated fats.

Trans-fats occur to a small extent in nature but the largest source comes from a process called hydrogenation. This process is used to improve the shelf life of vegetable oils.

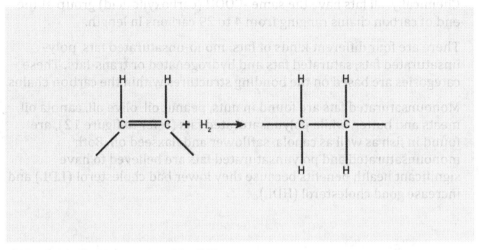

Figure 13. Hydrogenation Process

Trans-fats are the unhealthiest fat and have been linked to an increase in cholesterol as well as to cardiovascular disease.[11]

Other than advocating the avoidance of trans-fats, the Fast Tract Diet does not specifically limit fats as they don't contribute to bacterial overgrowth and resulting inflammation and symptoms.

Other Essential "Ingredients"

Now let's look at some of the other elements of our diet that are required for good health. Along with proteins and fats, our bodies require water, vitamins, minerals, specific types of essential fatty acids, and amino acids. (Carbohydrates are not technically a nutritional requirement, since fats can meet all of our energy requirements.)

Water

Water is the most important single metabolic requirement we have. We need water to break down and metabolize every food group; as well as for transporting nutrients and removing waste from around the body. Water is also critical for maintaining body temperature, osmotic balance (controlling salt and other electrolyte concentrations), blood pressure and normal bowel and bladder functions. Lack of water is one of the surest ways to degrade a wide range of normal bodily functions.

Vitamins

Vitamins are required for a variety of digestive and cellular processes, primarily as co-enzymes (helper molecules for enzymes). Essential vitamins include vitamins A (retinol), Bp (choline), B1 (thiamine), B2 (riboflavin), B3 (niacin), B5 (pantothenic acid), B6 (pyridoxine), B7 (biotin), B9 (folic acid), B10 (p-aminobenzoic acid), B12 (cobalamine), C (ascorbic acid), D (calciferol), E (tocopherol) and K (naphthoquinone). The vitamins present in a balanced diet are usually sufficient for our purposes, taking a daily multivitamin ensures an ample supply of needed vitamins.

Minerals

Minerals are also required for enzymes to function; giving bones their strength, and cells the ability to regulate fluid levels. Key minerals include; calcium, chloride, magnesium, phosphorus, potassium, sodium and sulfur. Other minerals such as copper, chromium, iodine, iron, manganese molybdenum selenium, zinc and possibly boron, nickel, tin, silicon and vanadium are required in trace amounts. Minerals are generally plentiful in our diet or in the water we drink, but to be on the safe side you can take a daily multivitamin that also contains minerals.

Omega-3 and Omega-6 Fatty Acids

Essential polyunsaturated fatty acids (PUFAs) include omega-3 and omega-6 fatty acids. Our bodies cannot manufacture these compounds, so you must supply them in your diet. Most diets are rich in omega-6 fatty acids; but omega-3 fatty acids are present in fewer foods. Good sources of omega-3 fatty acids include: alpha-linolenic acid from flaxseed oil, canola or walnut oil; and fish oil-based eicosapentaenoic acid (EPA) and docosahexaenoic acid (DHA) found in fish (fish get EPA and DHA from eating algae). Alpha-linolenic acid can be converted into EPA and DHA in the body though not at 100 percent efficiency. So it's a good idea to eat fatty fish such as mackerel, trout, sardines, tuna, or salmon a few times per week, or take a fish oil supplement. [12]

Amino Acids

Essential amino acids include isoleucine, lysine, leucine, methionine, phenylalanine, threonine, tryptophan and valine, but also histidine and arginine in children.

Deficiencies in essential amino acids are very rare. Animal-based protein contains all of the essential amino acids. Even though some plant-based proteins are deficient in amino acids such as lysine, methionine or tryptophan, consuming a variety of plant protein sources can easily give you an adequate supply of all essential amino acids.

Inessential "Ingredients": Sweeteners

Sweeteners aren't essential like other "foods" in this chapter, but they are used by almost everyone in some form every day.

Natural Sweeteners

The most common sweetener is sucrose or table sugar. Sucrose is a disaccharide (meaning it's composed of two sugar molecules stuck together) containing equal amounts of glucose and fructose. Sucrose is not used in the recipes in this book because it contains 50 percent fructose, which can be difficult for some people to absorb (more on this later). The same goes for high fructose corn syrup, which generally contains more fructose than glucose, and honey, which has approximately the same ratio of glucose to fructose as sucrose. Most people can tolerate small amounts of sucrose and honey, but moderation is the key.

Fructose itself is also used as a common sweetener in many foods, snacks and desserts and is almost twice as sweet as sucrose or honey. I would advise strictly limiting fructose as it is very difficult to absorb, particularly in the absence of glucose. This can be challenging given the widespread use of this sweetener.

Sugar alcohols, also known as polyols, represent a group of non-carbohydrate sweeteners. Sugar alcohols include sorbitol, mannitol, xylitol, lactitol, isomalt, erythritol, and maltitol. In general, sugar alcohols are poorly absorbed, so they don't raise insulin levels much, but can be fermented by gut bacteria, potentially causing diarrhea, gas, bloating and reflux. For this reason, sugar alcohols should be avoided. (See chapter 7 for more information on sugar alcohols.)

Artificial Sweeteners

There are several artificial sweeteners on the market that provide alternatives for people who want to avoid sweeteners that contain fructose. Artificial sweeteners generally have no carbohydrates and zero calories but simply taste sweet. Sucralose (Splenda) is the most popular followed by aspartame (Equal and NutraSweet), stevia (SweetLeaf, Truvia and Stevia Blend), and saccharin.

Sucralose (Splenda) was approved for use in the US in 1998. Sucralose is similar in many ways to sucrose, but has been chemically modified so that it is not digestible — by people *or* bacteria. This property makes it ideal for people with digestive problems including GERD. Sucralose is also stable when heated, so can be used for baking or in other hot recipes. Sucralose, which has an excellent safety record, has been used as a sweetener for most of the recipes in this book.

Equal and NutraSweet both contain aspartame which was approved by the FDA in 1981. The sweetener can break down when exposed to heat so is not good for baking. Aspartame may also cause mild headaches and other side effects in some people. In general, I would avoid this sweetener in favor of sucralose. Also, people who have the rare genetic condition known as phenylketonuria must avoid aspartame because it contains the amino acid phenylalanine.

Stevia marketed as SweetLeaf, Truvia and Stevia Blend, is a natural sweetener that comes from the leaves of the South American plant *Stevia rebaudiana*. This sweetener has been used for decades in other countries but only recently has found its way into the US market. I haven't used this sweetener myself, but the sources I checked seem to indicate it has a relatively good safety record. Like sucralose, stevia is heat stable and can be used in cooking.

There is only one problem with stevia: All of the brands I checked, including Stevia Blend, SweetLeaf and Truvia, also contain sugar alcohol and, in the case of Stevia Blend, fructose oligosaccharide as ingredients. Both of these substances are not absorbed by the small intestine and are highly fermentable by gut bacteria. For this reason, these sweeteners should be avoided completely.

Saccharin (Sweet'N Low) is another artificial sweetener that contains just under one gram of dextrose (glucose) as one of its ingredients. Based on testing in rats in the sixties, the sweetener was thought to cause cancer, leading the FDA to require a warning on the product, the cancer fears were determined to be unfounded in humans and the warnings were removed in 2001. Despite its bitter aftertaste, many people prefer it to other sweeteners. Like aspartame, saccharin is not stable when heated and cannot be used for baking.

Now that you have a better idea of just what "raw materials" your digestive system has to deal with, we can take the next step in understanding digestion: looking into how your body metabolizes all of these different foods.

Chapter 3: Healthy Digestion

Next, I'd like to give you a simplified look at how the digestive process is supposed to work. It's much easier to understand how and why GERD develops if you know the basics of how your digestive tract is supposed to act.

Before your body can get the nutrition it needs from the three food groups described in the previous chapter, they must be broken down into their basic "building blocks" through the process of digestion:

> *Carbohydrates are broken down to monosaccharides*

> *Proteins are broken down to amino acids*

> *Fats are broken down to fatty acids*

Once broken down, they can be absorbed into the blood stream and available for use by the cells in our body or stored as glycogen or fat.

First, let's take a step-by-step look at the pathway food takes as it is processed by your digestive system:

The Digestive Process

Mouth

Your digestive system starts working even before you take a bite of food. Your senses — primarily smell and taste — trigger the release of saliva and enzymes to prepare your digestive system to process the food.

As soon as you take a bite, your chewing helps break the food up into smaller digestible pieces. At the same time, six salivary glands in your mouth release saliva to help lubricate and liquefy the food. Saliva also contains the enzyme amylase, which begins breaking the chemical bonds between the sugar molecules that hold complex carbohydrates together. When you swallow, rings of muscles around the esophagus push the food towards your stomach through a coordinated wave of contractions, known as peristalsis. At the lower end of the esophagus, a group of muscles collectively referred to as the lower esophageal sphincter (or LES) relax, letting the food pass into your stomach.

Stomach

By the time the food arrives in your stomach, your body has responded to the smell and taste of the food by releasing histamine. This stimulates the specialized "parietal" cells lining the stomach to produce hydrochloric acid (HCl). The HCl creates an extremely acidic environment that kills bacteria in the food, denatures (unfolds) proteins, and activates the enzyme pepsin, which breaks large proteins into smaller molecules (polypeptides). The stomach protects itself from the acid by producing a coating of mucus. The stomach also produces the enzyme lipase, which helps breakdown fats into triglycerides.

To churn the food together with stomach acid and enzymes, muscles contained in wall of the stomach contract in a coordinated fashion. After a few hours, the partially digested food, called chyme, consists of a mixture of polypeptides (partially broken down protein), polysaccharides (partially digested carbohydrates) and triglycerides (partially broken down fats). The chyme is released from the stomach through the pyloric sphincter, another ring of muscles, to the duodenum, which is the first part of the small intestine.

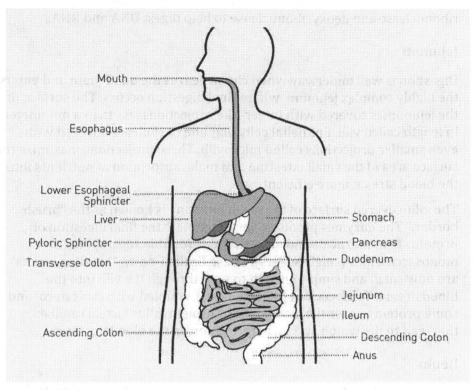

Figure 14. Human Digestive Tract

The diagram is labeled as follows:

- Mouth
- Esophagus
- Lower Esophageal Sphincter
- Liver
- Pyloric Sphincter
- Transverse Colon
- Ascending Colon
- Stomach
- Pancreas
- Duodenum
- Jejunum
- Ileum
- Descending Colon
- Anus

Small Intestine

The small intestine is approximately 20 feet long and divided into three sections (in this order): the duodenum, jejunum and ileum. The two main purposes of the small intestine are to complete the digestive process started in the stomach, and then absorb the digested nutrients into the blood.

Duodenum

As chyme enters your duodenum, your pancreas releases bicarbonate to neutralize the stomach acid. It also produces additional enzymes, including amylase for polysaccharide digestion, proteases and elastase for peptide digestion, and lipase for triglyceride digestion. Bile, produced in the liver and stored in the gall bladder, is released to help with the breakdown and absorption of triglycerides. The pancreas also produces ribonuclease and deoxyribonuclease to help digest DNA and RNA.

Jejunum

Digestion is well underway when chyme leaves the duodenum and enters the highly complex jejunum, where final digestion occurs. The surface of the jejunum is covered with finger-like projections less than a millimeter in length called villi. Epithelial cells that line the villi are covered with even smaller projections called microvilli. These projections maximize the surface area of the small intestine and make absorption of nutrients into the blood stream more efficient.

The villi-covered surface of the small intestine is known as the "brush border." The enzymes produced here complete the final digestion of proteins to amino acids and disaccharides (double sugars) into monosaccharides (single sugars). These broken-down "building blocks" are now small and simple enough to pass through the villi into the bloodstream. Triglycerides (digested fats), coupled with cholesterol and some proteins, enter the bloodstream through villus lacteal capillaries that lead to the lymph system before entering the bloodstream.

Ileum

Chyme, which at this point contains only undigested food and the by-products of digestion, eventually enters the third part of the small intestine, the ileum, where water, some vitamins and bile salts (used to break down fats) are absorbed. Both water and bile salts are recycled as part of the overall digestive process. At this point the primary digestion and nutrient absorption process is complete. The leftover chyme leaves the small intestine via the ileocecal valve and enters the large intestine.

The number of intestinal bacteria steadily increases towards the last part of the small intestine. Peristalsis, intestinal immunity, and efficient absorption of nutrients help keep these bacterial populations in check. Intestinal bacteria play a key role in the development of GERD, and will be looked at in more detail a little later in this book.

Large Intestine (or Colon)

Residual material entering the colon has been depleted of many nutrients but still contains resistant starch, fiber and some protein that escaped digestion in the small intestine. As this material moves through the colon, bacteria ferment the remaining starch, protein and much of the fiber.

Water and electrolytes (salts) are removed and recycled and the stool is formed and stored until a bowel movement occurs.

By comparison with the small intestine, the human large intestine is a breeding ground for bacteria. On average, it contains over 100 trillion microorganisms representing over 500 different species. Humans and gut bacteria have evolved together over millions of years. The result is a mutually beneficial relationship: They live on nutrients in our diet that we are unable to digest and would otherwise be wasted. In exchange, bacteria produce some vitamins and other nutrients that nourish our own cells. Bacteria allow us to use food up to 30 percent more efficiently than we could without them. (This is about the same as boosting the gas mileage in your car from 20 miles per gallon to 26 miles per gallon.)

Healthy intestinal bacteria also compete with and protect us from germs that can cause diseases. Bacteria represent the bulk of intestinal organisms, though some protozoa, fungi and other tiny life-forms reside here as well.

The Role of Bacteria in Digestion

Most people know that bacteria play some role in the digestive process, but most people are surprised by just how important this role is. Understanding how our gut bacterial populations work is key to understanding the symptoms and proper treatment of GERD.

Bacteria in the Small Intestine

Bacteria most common to the small intestine include *Lactobacillus, Enterococcus, Staphylococcus,* and *Streptococcus* species, with the most prevalent type being *Lactobacillus.*

The *Lactobacillus* species play a key role in the small intestine. The *Lactobacillus* species, including *Lactobacillus acidophilus* (present in yogurt), ferment small amounts of unabsorbed sugars such as lactose and other disaccharides to produce lactic acid.

Outside the digestive process, lactic acid is a common commercial preservative used to preserve food; just as naturally made lactic acid helps yogurt last a long time in the refrigerator. Inside the small intestine, it maintains an acidic environment that is unfavorable to the many "unhealthy" bacteria.

Lactobacillus acidophilus and several related species present in the small intestine are known as homolactic fermenters. These types of bacteria produce predominantly one end produce, lactic acid. Unlike most other bacteria, homolactic fermenters do not produce gaseous end products. This trait is desirable and likely contributes to the success of *Lactobacillus acidophilus* as a probiotic.

Other (heterolactic) bacteria break down starch and sugars to produce a wide variety of end products including lactic, acetic, propionic and butyric acids, but they also produce gases such as carbon dioxide, hydrogen, and sometimes methane. These gases can cause a number of unpleasant symptoms as well as acid reflux.

Bacteria in the Large Intestine

Bacteria common to the large intestine include *Bifidobacteria, Bacteroides, Actinocyces, Fusobacteria, E. coli, Enterocci, Streptococci, Clostridia, Corynebacteri, Enterobacter, Proteus, Klebsiella, Propionibacteria*, as well as *Lactobacilli* and several hundred less common species.

For the most part, we live in mutually beneficial harmony with these highly specialized single-celled creatures for our entire lives. As noted above, they consume food that we fail to digest and, in return, producing high-energy short-chain fatty acids that our cells can use for energy; vitamins, such as biotin, folate and vitamin K; and out-compete disease-causing bacteria like *C. diff*, helping to maintain normal gut function and stimulating our own immunity.

The foods that we either can't digest or digest poorly usually end up in the colon. These include plant fibers such as cellulose and pectin, oligosaccharides stachyose and raffinose as well as the starch amylose and even sugars like fructose and lactose. Some bacteria in the colon can even break down cellulose and hemicellulose fiber. Bacteria that are able to break down these "waste products" clearly have a competitive advantage.

The predominance of *Bifidobacteria* and *Bacteroides* in the large intestine is no accident. These bacteria have adapted perfectly to the human large intestine with their ability to break down complex and difficult to digest polysaccharides including amylose starch as well as the oligosaccharides stachyose and raffinose.

As an example of how specialized these bacteria have become, *Bifidibacteria* have the ability to rapidly degrade oligosaccharides using a unique metabolic pathway called the "bifid shunt." Amazingly, *Bifidobacteria* are able to use the oligosaccharides stachyose and raffinose (that we can't digest) more efficiently than they can use simple glucose.[13]

The bacteria living in our colons have adapted to life without oxygen — as there is none in the large intestine. That means that these anaerobic bacteria depend on the process of fermentation (deriving energy from nutrients in the absence of oxygen) to survive.

As part of fermentation, bacteria collectively secrete a large array of enzymes that break down the tough remaining nutrients to produce energy and the raw materials they need for their own existence and reproduction. As part of the process, they also produce lactic acid, acetic acid, propionic acid, ethanol and butyric acid as well as the gases hydrogen, carbon dioxide and sometimes methane.

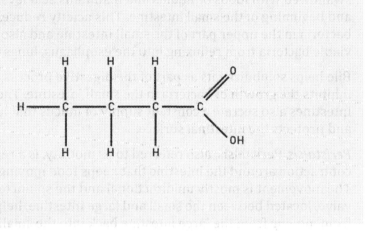

Figure 15. Butyric Acid

This fermentation process, as it turns out, is one of the key elements in the development of GERD. Most people aren't even aware of its existence, yet it plays a critical role in their quality of life!

A Healthy Balance

As in most biological or physiological processes, the key to health is maintaining a healthy balance between different aspects of the process.

For example, while the large intestine can deal with huge numbers (trillions) of bacteria, the small intestine can't. Unfortunately, there's a direct physical link between the two — the ileocecal valve! Since the small intestine houses the crucial digestive and absorptive machinery we need to maintain our nutrition, it's essential that the small intestine is protected against potential invasion and overpopulation by bacteria from the large intestine (SIBO).[14]

To maintain digestive health, then, the body must ensure that the bulk of bacterial fermentation occurs in the large intestine and limit fermentation in the small intestine. Besides maintaining a population of friendly, protective bacteria, the small intestine has a number of other defenses that protect it and the digestive process against these harmful bacteria.

These include:

Stomach acid, bile and mucous secretions. Stomach acid kills most bacteria swallowed with foods or liquids and maintains acid levels in the stomach and beginning of the small intestine. This acidity reduces the number of bacteria in the upper part of the small intestine and also helps prevent viable bacteria from refluxing into the esophagus, lungs or sinuses.

Bile helps solubilize fats as part of the digestive process, but it also inhibits the growth of bacteria in the small intestine. The stomach and intestines also secrete a constant supply of mucus that lubricates, coats and protects the intestinal surface.

Peristalsis. Peristalsis, also referred to as motility, is a regular muscular contraction around the intestine that keeps food moving through the gut. The movement is mostly unidirectional and the sphincter-shaped ileocecal valve, located between the small and large intestine, helps keep bacteria from moving from the large intestine back into the small intestine. This constant movement of food during digestion also limits the amount and type of bacterial fermentation in the small intestine.

Efficient digestion and absorption of carbohydrates. When carbohydrates are broken down and fully absorbed they leave the small intestine and enter the blood stream as glucose. The more efficient this process is, the less "leftover" fuel there is for small intestinal bacterial growth.

Immune surveillance. The final layer of protection is active immune surveillance. Specific antimicrobial mucin proteins and alpha defensin peptides (peptides are small proteins) are produced by the intestinal epithelial cells to prevent foreign bacteria from invading. Antibodies such as IgA and IgM are produced in response to specific identifying proteins on the surface of bacteria. Antibodies identify and protect friendly bacteria and help attack threatening bacteria.

SIBO and GERD get their start when this balance starts to fall apart. One of the goals of the Fast Tract Diet is to show you what you can do to help your body maintain the integrity and balance of your digestive process.

Chapter 4: The True Cause of GERD

As mentioned previously, the conventional wisdom states that GERD is caused by weakness, relaxation or damage to the lower esophageal sphincter (or LES). While LES weakness can certainly be a part of the problem, it is much more likely that GERD and related digestive conditions are caused by an imbalance in the growth of bacterial populations in our intestines.

Let's look at what happens when a healthy digestive system begins to lose its "balance."

The Role of SIBO

To understand how bacterial imbalance causes GERD, we first have to look at a related medical condition: SIBO, or Small Intestinal Bacterial Overgrowth.

SIBO is defined as the presence of an abnormally high number of bacteria (more than 100,000 bacteria per milliliter) in the upper part of the small intestine. At this level, the normally harmless bacteria that live in our gut can become harmful. They begin to produce toxins, enzymes, short-chain fatty acids and intestinal gases, including hydrogen, methane, and carbon dioxide that can disrupt digestion, cause intense physical discomfort and even damage the small intestine.

The symptoms of SIBO include abdominal pain or cramps, diarrhea, constipation, gas, bloating, acid reflux (the focus of this book), flatulence, nausea, dehydration and fatigue. More severe symptoms related to SIBO can include weight loss and "failure to thrive," steatorrhea (the body's failure to digest fats), anemia, bleeding or bruising, night blindness, bone pain and fractures, leaky gut syndrome, and autoimmune reactions, among others.

Symptoms such as vomiting, constant diarrhea, fever or blood in the stool are indicators of even more serious illness and should be evaluated by your doctor as soon as possible.

These symptoms will vary from one individual to another and may not be present at all times. Symptoms might go away for one month, only to return the next. However, SIBO is likely to recur until the underlying causes of the bacterial overgrowth are corrected. The only sure way to relieve these symptoms is to bring the balance of bacteria growth between the small and large intestines back under control.

What Causes SIBO?

The bacteria associated with SIBO originate from our own intestines; particularly the large intestine. Bacterial types isolated from the small intestine of people with SIBO include: *Streptococcus*, *Staphylococcus*, and *Lactobacillus* — all generally associated with the small intestine; and *E. coli*, *Micrococcus*, *Klebsiella*, *Proteus*, *Bacteriodes*, *Clostridium*, *Veillonella*, *Fusobacterium* and *Peptostreptococcus* — all generally associated with the large intestine.[15]

SIBO is tightly linked to carbohydrate malabsorption — in which gut bacteria use excess carbohydrates left over when digestion is incomplete to grow and multiply. In the words of Elaine Gottschall, the conditions are parts of a "Vicious Cycle" that plays out in our small intestine. Bacteria feed on unabsorbed carbohydrates, grow and produce acids, gasses, toxins, enzymes, and assorted waste products that cause an inflammatory reaction in our digestive tract.

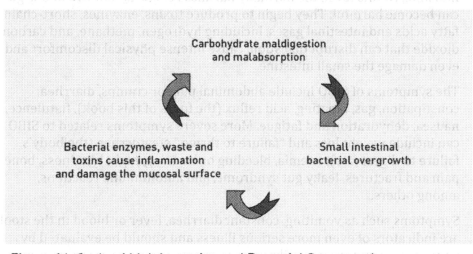

Figure 16. Cycle of Malabsorption and Bacterial Overgrowth

The inflammatory reaction injures the mucosal lining of the small intestine. The injured cells on the mucosal surface are unable to complete the breakdown and absorption of food. This leads to a higher level of malabsorbed carbohydrates, feeding the overgrowth of even more bacteria. This vicious cycle is played out over and over again in the small intestines all over the world.

How Does SIBO Cause GERD?

One of the key products of bacterial overgrowth is gas, usually carbon dioxide, hydrogen, and in some people, methane. This gas raises the pressure level in the small intestine and stomach that I believe can actually drive the reflux of viscous stomach contents into the esophagus.

These refluxed stomach contents contain acid, digestive enzymes, bile and even bacteria. The burning sensation, or heartburn, that most people with GERD feel is a direct result of stomach acid on the unprotected esophagus. In some cases the stomach acid, digestive enzymes and bacteria are refluxed beyond the esophagus and reach the lungs and sinuses, causing a variety of new symptoms and creating more serious health problems — including pneumonia and potentially contributing to asthma.

Can this bacterial fermentation really create enough (gas) pressure in the digestive system to cause acid reflux? It certainly can! Years ago, as a research scientist, I routinely grew bacterial cultures of *E. coli*, *Bacteroides fragilis* and other intestinal bacteria in the laboratory.

The growth media we used contained a carbohydrate source (usually glucose) because gut bacteria like to consume carbohydrates for energy. I was amazed at the amount of gas that most strains could produce. As little as thirty grams (the weight of six nickels) of carbohydrate is enough to allow bacteria to produce ten liters of hydrogen gas. (Intestinal bacteria can create so much flammable gas that there have been well-documented cases of explosions during intestinal surgery.[16])

If bacterial overgrowth can cause that much gas pressure, it can certainly drive acid reflux into the esophagus.

The Scientific Evidence That SIBO Causes GERD

This is a fundamental change in the way we understand GERD, with critical implications for treatment protocols, and I don't expect you — or the medical community — to just take my word for it. Fortunately, the scientific evidence for this connection has been building over the past decade.

My research has uncovered five distinct points of evidence which convinced me that poor carbohydrate absorption (or malabsorption) coupled with SIBO may be the ultimate cause of acid reflux.

1. *Restricting the growth of intestinal bacteria, whether by limiting carbohydrate intake or treating with antibiotics, reduces the symptoms of GERD, including reflux and gas pressure.*

Reducing dietary carbohydrates is effective at relieving GERD symptoms and reducing esophageal acid exposure.[17] I believe this is because intestinal bacteria are denied fuel, which limits their growth and their ability to produce intestinal gas. The Fast Tract Diet takes this a step further specifically limiting the most difficult to digest carbs. The data from the Fast Tract Diet clinical study (Chapter 1) provided evidence for the effectiveness of this approach.

Treatment of GERD patients with the antibiotic erythromycin was shown to decrease reflux and increase apparent LES pressure. The authors suggested that the antibiotic strengthened the lower esophageal sphincter (LES).[18] But how can an antibiotic tighten these muscles? It seems much more likely that the antibiotic is limiting the growth of the gut microbial population. Fewer bacteria mean less fermentation, less gas and less reflux.

In another study, antibiotics reduced GERD symptoms, as well as esophageal acid exposure and the concentration of bile acids in fluid removed from the lungs of lung transplant patients. [19] The effect of the antibiotics on preventing digestive fluids from reaching the esophagus and even the lungs indicates the drug is affecting a single underlying process. In this case, the antibiotics are most likely reducing bacterial activity and, as a result, reflux, the symptoms of GERD and lung damage in the transplant patients studied.

2. *Carbohydrate malabsorption and GERD can be created experimentally.*

Ingesting the carbohydrate fructose oligosaccharide, which is indigestible by humans, but fermentable by bacteria, produces intestinal gas and GERD symptoms.[20] The authors noted an increase in the Transient Lower Esophageal Sphincter Relaxations (TLESRs). In other words, the LES opened more as if it was relaxing. I believe the "lower esophageal sphincter relaxations" described by the authors actually represent the LES being "forced" open by gas pressure.

Consuming fructose oligosaccharide (FOS) creates 100% malabsorption. The fermentation of FOS by gut bacteria creates enough gas to pressurize the small intestine and stomach and force open the LES — causing reflux and heartburn.

3. GERD is associated with increased gas pressure in the stomach.

People with GERD have been shown to have increased gas pressure in their stomach and belch more frequently.[21] This is consistent with the idea that gas produced by bacteria in the small intestine can create gas pressure, belching, and other GERD symptoms. The only difference between belching and acid reflux is that the gas pushes stomach contents into the esophagus in the latter case and escapes on its own in the former. Drinking lots of water can help, as less viscous stomach contents are more likely to allow belching before reflux.

Also, fundoplication surgery is linked to new symptoms in a significant number of GERD patients. The new symptoms include excessive gas and bloating.[22] The procedure is aimed at preventing reflux by tightening the LES muscles surgically, but the side effects are indicative of trapped stomach and intestinal gas as would be expected with uncontrolled malabsorption, and excessive bacterial fermentation.

4. Health conditions associated with malabsorption and SIBO are linked to GERD.

Approximately eighty percent of people with cystic fibrosis (CF) also have GERD. This compares to less than twenty percent in the general population.[23] People with CF also exhibit well-documented carbohydrate malabsorption and bacterial overgrowth. CF can play a role in the development of GERD since the CF patients often have blockage of the pancreatic ducts by thick mucous which blocks the release of the enzyme pancreatic amylase limiting carbohydrate digestion and absorption, leading to a higher level of carbohydrates available to gut bacteria. In GERD sufferers that don't have CF, amylase release isn't blocked, but there is still an oversupply of difficult to digest carbohydrates available to induce reflux.

The prevalence of GERD in IBS patients (39%) and IBS in GERD patients (49%) is much higher than the prevalence of GERD (19%) or IBS (12%) in the general population.[24] IBS has been clearly linked to small intestinal bacterial overgrowth by hydrogen breath testing and, like GERD, has been treated successfully with carbohydrate restriction as well as antibiotics.[25] This evidence is consistent with SIBO playing a role in both conditions.

Obesity is associated with GERD and carbohydrate restriction improves

GERD symptoms and reduces esophageal acid exposure in these patients whether or not they lose weight.[26] Obese individuals generally consume more food, especially carbohydrates, which I believe leads to malabsorption, SIBO, and reflux.

5. SIBO has been detected in GERD patients.

Half of GERD patients taking PPI drugs showed evidence of SIBO by glucose breath testing (see section below on breath testing to detect SIBO) compared to only 25% of IBS patients not taking PPIs.[27] Eighty-seven to ninety percent of SIBO-positive patients (with GERD or IBS) showed improvement after antibiotic treatment. I believe the SIBO-positive results in both groups would have been even higher if the study employed the lactulose breath test instead of the glucose breath test.

Lactulose is not digested or absorbed in the small intestine and can detect bacteria (fermenting the lactulose and producing hydrogen) throughout the entire length of the small intestine. Glucose is rapidly absorbed in the first part of the small intestine and will only detect bacteria if they are present in this region. Mark Pimentel found that 78 percent of IBS patients tested at the Cedars-Sinai Medical Center had SIBO as indicated by a positive lactulose test.[28]

In my opinion, the very name "Gastrointestinal Esophageal Reflux Disease" is misleading. I don't believe GERD is a "disease" at all, but rather a condition brought about by the marketing of, and easy access to, large quantities of foods containing difficult-to-digest carbohydrates or a symptom of other underlying conditions that promote SIBO.

Diagnosing SIBO in people with GERD

Mainstream medicine does not pursue a diagnostic or treatment strategy based on SIBO for people suffering from GERD. The reason is because my research linking GERD with bacterial overgrowth is new and clinical research in this area is limited.

Once the diagnosis of GERD has been established, generally based on chronic heartburn or other reflux-related symptoms, most medical doctors prescribe treatment with acid-reducing medicines. PPIs are the most powerful acid-reducing meds and are also the most frequently prescribed. To determine if your GERD symptoms are related to bacterial overgrowth you could ask your health care provider to test you for the presence of SIBO. (Because my research linking GERD with bacterial overgrowth is still considered theoretical, this testing may not be covered by your insurance.)

Diagnostic test methods for SIBO are far from perfect. You may be better off just trying the Fast Tract Diet, which is aimed treating SIBO, and see if it relieves your symptoms.

If you are interested in getting tested, there are two basic tests for SIBO: bacterial culture and hydrogen breath testing.

Bacterial Culture Testing

The most definitive test for small intestinal bacterial overgrowth is to actually take a sample of the small intestine contents, culture the sample in a diagnostic microbiology laboratory, and determine the types and concentration of bacteria present. More than one hundred thousand bacteria per milliliter indicates overgrowth.

The bacterial culture method is really the "gold standard" for this diagnosis, but it is an invasive technique, requiring significant expertise both on the part of the clinician as well as the laboratory analyzing the samples. Getting accurate results can be challenging, due to the difficulty of obtaining a sample from the small intestine, protecting it from contamination, transporting the sample to the lab, and analyzing the sample before the bacterial count changes.

Even then, the results don't tell you anything about the types of bacteria present. That would require further bacteriological typing. Also, the majority of organisms present in the sample are anaerobic, meaning they cannot grow in the presence of air. Special culturing techniques are needed to detect and identify anaerobic bacteria. And, since a large number of intestinal bacteria simply don't grow in culture, some bacteria would still go undetected. In practical terms, this method is almost never used.

Hydrogen Breath Testing

Hydrogen breath testing (sometimes referred to as lactulose breath testing) is more commonly used to detect SIBO. Following an overnight fast, a lactulose sugar solution is given to the patient orally after which breath samples are taken (the patient breaths into a sampling device) each 15 minutes over a three-hour period, and then analyzed for the concentration of hydrogen.

Lactulose is a sugar that cannot be digested by humans (in medical terms, lactulose is 100% *malabsorbed*) so it travels through the small and then large intestine until it encounters bacteria. Many bacteria, on the other hand, *can* break down and utilize lactulose-producing hydrogen as a waste product.

Some of this hydrogen is absorbed into the blood stream and released from the lungs where it shows up in the breath sample. Since human metabolism does not generate hydrogen, any hydrogen detected has to come from bacteria. The hydrogen measurements from the breath samples are used to create a plot or graph of hydrogen released over the entire three hours.

Healthy people are relatively free of bacteria in the early part of the small intestine. Their test results typically show a single large peak of hydrogen in breath samples taken about 2 hours after the lactulose solution is given, representing fermentation of the lactulose by bacteria in the large intestine. Test results for people with SIBO will show hydrogen concentrations of 20 or more parts per million in samples collected within 90 minutes or less after the lactulose solution is consumed,[29] representing fermentation of the lactulose by bacteria in the small intestine. This pattern is a strong indication of the presence of SIBO.

One of the challenges in gaining wider acceptance for the use of hydrogen breath testing is the need for standardization of the breath testing technique. Some tests replace lactulose with glucose and as a result can only detect SIBO in the earliest part of the small intestine. Practitioners are also challenged by the differences between analyses at different labs, and the lack of definitive studies comparing the breath test results to microbiological culture methods. More information is needed before we can gauge the sensitivity (how much SIBO must be present to detect it?) and specificity (are some of the results falsely positive?) of the method.

Hydrogen Breath Testing for Individual Carbohydrates

Hydrogen breath testing can also be used to detect the malabsorption of individual sugars other than lactulose.[30]

This diagnostic tool is based on the fact that digested and absorbed sugars will enter the blood stream and not be available for intestinal fermentation. (And, therefore, testing will not reveal a hydrogen peak.) Unabsorbed or poorly absorbed sugars will remain in the intestine and become fermented, releasing hydrogen (demonstrating a hydrogen peak and a positive test for specific sugar malabsorption). This test has even been used to detect the malabsorption of starch.

To conduct this test, the patient drinks a solution containing the suspect carbohydrate, such as lactose, fructose or other carbohydrate. The test administrator will measure the amount of hydrogen present in breath samples over a three-hour period.

Any sugar that is unabsorbed will be consumed by bacteria in the small intestine as well as the large intestine. How soon hydrogen is detected indicates whether the patient has SIBO (an early hydrogen signal indicates bacterial growth in the upper small intestine) or not (a late hydrogen signal indicates fermentation by bacteria in the large intestine) as well as whether or not the specific sugar has been digested and absorbed into the blood stream (and is therefore unavailable for bacterial consumption).

Future Trends in Treating SIBO

The complexity of intestinal microflora and its importance in human health is just beginning to be fully recognized. No less than thirty disease conditions involve an out-of-balance gut *microbiota* (the gut microbe population as a whole).

My research supports the view that limiting malabsorption and addressing underlying conditions that promote SIBO can treat many digestive conditions, but there is also a more radical approach.

Can the restoration of a "normal" or more balanced population of gut microbes cure or improve these diseases and conditions? Research in this area is still limited. Most of the work has focused on the treatment of C diff infections where conventional treatments have failed. But so far, the answer seems to be, "yes."

Replacing the entire microflora of someone suffering a digestive illness with the microflora of a healthy person may be the best way to jump start recovery from intestinal infections and possibly other SIBO related conditions.

Amazing as this sounds (and maybe a little unsettling to some), this treatment is called fecal bacteriotherapy. It is common in veterinary medicine and is now being performed successfully in humans. The sick person is treated with antibiotics and bowel lavage followed by the introduction of a fecal suspension (containing gut bacteria) from a healthy donor prescreened for a variety of illnesses and pathogens.

Fecal bacteriotherapy has been used to treat close to two hundred

43

patients suffering from *C diff* (some critically ill) with a success rate of greater than 90 percent.[31] Encouraging results have also been obtained in the treatment of patients with inflammatory bowel disease, IBS, and chronic constipation.[32]

More work needs to be done to understand the exactly how this treatment works, but two things are clear. The patient responses are long lasting (years in some cases), and the transplanted microorganisms are able to survive and persist in the recipients. In one case, transplanted microbes were recovered 24 weeks after the procedure.[33] Longer times were not tested in the study. Who knows? One day fecal transplantation could be used to treat GERD.

My goal in this chapter was to show you the evidence linking poor carbohydrate absorption to SIBO to GERD. In the chapters that follow, we'll look at what the implications are for treating GERD, and offer the details of the Fast Tract Diet— specifically designed to make it easier for you to reduce or eliminate your symptom.

Chapter 5: Better Treatments for GERD

Now that we've taken a closer look at the relationship between poor digestion, malabsorption, SIBO, and GERD, we're going to look at how to use this knowledge. Our new understanding of how GERD develops offers some promising avenues for developing more effective treatments. First, though, let's take a quick look at some of the approaches that have not worked out.

Trigger Food Diets

As discussed earlier, current diet treatments for GERD are based on the misconception that trigger foods cause the relaxation of the lower esophageal sphincter. Many "trigger" foods contain the same difficult-to-digest carbohydrates that feed SIBO.

The biggest offenders? Fructose, including high-fructose corn syrup, lactose, sucrose (which is one-half fructose), resistant starch and fiber. One or more of these carbohydrate types inevitably are found in trigger foods:

Fried foods are often breaded or coated with wheat-based flour, which is high in resistant starch. French fries are made from potatoes. Most varieties of potatoes contain high amounts of resistant starch. Many fruits contain high amounts of fructose, and many dairy products contain lactose. Coffee is often times consumed sweetened with table sugar (sucrose) or milk that contains lactose. Wines that are sweet contain significant amounts of sugars, as do most carbonated beverages. Beer also contains resistant starch. Chocolate contains sucrose and is high in fiber. Spices can irritate the esophagus, but are not a "cause" of acid reflux.

The problem is that most trigger-food diets fail to limit *all* of the difficult-to-digest carbohydrates that I believe are the real triggers for GERD. They also fail to employ practices, techniques, or digestive supplements that can minimize carbohydrate malabsorption.

As a result, most people on trigger-food diets continue to consume too many foods containing fructose, lactose, resistant starch, fiber, and sometimes, sugar alcohols, and continue to experience symptoms.

Proton Pump Inhibitors (PPI)

In chapter one, I discussed the side effects and health problems that have been associated with PPI drugs. To make matters worse, there is clear evidence that PPI drugs such as Nexium, Aciphex, Prilosec, Prevacid, and

Protonix are "addictive," because they create a significant "rebound effect" once you stop taking them.[34] Most people will actually experience worse reflux than they had before taking the drug.

In a brilliant study led by Christina Reimer at Copenhagen University in Denmark, 120 healthy subjects (without GERD) were divided into two groups. Sixty subjects were given Nexium for eight weeks then placebo for another four weeks while the remaining 60 subjects received placebo for the entire 12 weeks. Between weeks 9 and 12 (when the Nexium was stopped) 44% of the people who had been on the drug reported at least one GERD-related symptom while only 15% of the placebo group reported one or more symptoms. After 12 weeks, 21% of the Nexium group still reported at least one symptom of GERD while only 2% of the placebo group reported one or more symptoms.[35]

This amazing study showed that there is a rebound effect with these drugs whether or not you had GERD. The authors suggest that a phenomenon called drug-induced "rebound acid hyper-secretion" (RAHS) may be responsible, In other words, taking PPI drugs cause you to hyper-secrete stomach acid when the drug is removed.

I have another explanation that I think is more plausible. PPI drugs block the production of stomach acid. As we've discussed, lowered stomach acid can allow intestinal bacteria to grow in the upper small intestine and even the stomach — with the usual symptoms.[36]

The ironic conclusion is that PPIs can actually cause and perpetuate SIBO, what I believe to be the underlying cause of GERD. Luckily the effect will fade with the Fast Tract Diet as your stomach acid returns to normal and helps control SIBO.

If you are taking acid reducing medicines to control GERD-related symptoms and decide to try the Fast Tract Diet instead, talk to your doctor about gradually reducing the dosage of these medications to zero over a period of two to four weeks after starting the diet, using your symptoms as a guide.

Surgery

As discussed, fundoplication involves fastening part of the upper part of the stomach around the lower end of the esophagus to help close the LES against acid reflux. Unfortunately, a significant number of GERD patients who try this surgical approach develop new symptoms including excessive gas, bloating, diarrhea and abdominal pain. Also, the surgery is often not completely effective at preventing reflux symptoms and continued PPI therapy is required.

New Treatment Options

I have made the case that GERD is the result of bacterial overgrowth in the small intestine, fed by the poor absorption of carbohydrates that are difficult to digest.

The ratio of "bad" bacteria to "good" bacteria, the overall number of bacteria, and the rate of fermentation in the small intestine depends on many factors. Changes in any of these factors can disrupt the natural balance of the digestive system, creating conditions that allow bacteria to multiply excessively in the small intestine.

In order to successfully treat GERD, this destructive cycle of malabsorption, bacterial overgrowth, and inflammation must be disrupted. To achieve this goal, I have developed a three-part treatment strategy that represents the Fast Tract Diet System:

> *First, address any underlying condition(s) that promotes SIBO on a case-by-case basis (see chapter 6).*

> *Second, employ strategies and behaviors to minimize the malabsorption of difficult-to-digest carbohydrates (see chapters 6 and 7).*

> *Third, reduce the actual amount of difficult-to-digest carbohydrates with the Fast Tract Diet (see chapters 8 through 10).*

Chapter 6: Treating Underlying Factors

I am convinced that most people suffering from acid reflux simply consume too many difficult to digest carbs. For these individuals the Fast Tract Diet should result in rapid and complete relief of their symptoms. In some cases, there may be other contributing factors or underlying conditions that must also be identified and addressed to allow for a full recovery with the Fast Tract Diet. This chapter will help you and your health care provider develop a comprehensive treatment plan that addresses any other contributing conditions, should they exist.

Potential causes of SIBO (you likely suffer from one or more of these if you have heartburn) can be grouped into five categories:

Motility issues

Antibiotic use

Gastric (stomach) acid reduction

Immune impairment

Carbohydrate malabsorption

Motility Issues

Motility is based on the process of peristalsis — the coordination of intestinal muscles to keep food moving through the intestines. Problems with the muscles, nerves that control the muscles, intestinal scarring or blockages can all slow down motility. Changes in stool consistency, drugs, infections and SIBO itself can also alter motility. Both constipation and diarrhea are considered forms of dismotility.

Problems that can lead to alteration in motility include:

Structural defects of the intestine

Aging

Intestinal infections

Narrowing of the intestine due to scarring from Crohn's Disease or scleroderma

Surgical alteration of the intestine

Damage to the vagus nerve

Hypothyroidism

Drug Use

Damage to the vagus nerve from years of high blood sugar in type I and type II diabetes can result in prolonged gut transit times because the vagus nerve normally signals the muscles surrounding the intestine to contract. Similarly, intestinal motor dysfunction associated with hypothyroidism has been linked to SIBO.[37] Physical changes caused by surgery, infection, aging and scarring from Crohn's disease can also reduce peristalsis. Various drugs such as antidepressants, diuretics, pain medications or laxatives can also affect intestinal motility.

Regardless of the cause, slower peristalsis means longer gut transit times.[38] Bacteria in the small intestine have more time to break down and metabolize unabsorbed carbohydrates. As bacteria feed, they multiply and produce gas; waste products and cell debris than can damage the intestinal mucosal surface. One study showed that it took food on average 50 minutes longer to go from the mouth through the small intestine in people with SIBO, compared to people without SIBO.[39]

Treating Motility Problems

To end mild constipation, drink plenty of water (at least 8 glasses per day) and eat extra green vegetables. For more severe constipation, stool softeners, laxatives, or enemas may also help. These medicines should only be used occasionally, as overuse causes its own problems. Fiber supplements have also been used for constipation, but I would urge significant caution with these as they can make the problem worse. If severe constipation persists for several days, schedule a doctor's visit. Recent research has shown that constipation may indicate the intestinal overgrowth of methane-producing bacteria. This can be confirmed by methane breath testing. Since constipation is also a form of SIBO, the Fast Tract Diet should help with constipation.

Besides laxatives, other drugs such as antidepressants, diuretics and pain medications can influence motility. Changing medicines or reducing the dosage is an option you can explore with your doctor's help. Prescription pro-motility drugs do exist, but I would use them with caution, and discuss them with your doctor, because they have their own side effects, some serious.

Diarrhea caused by food poisoning, contaminated drinking water or intestinal infection is often self-limiting, but severe cases, especially involving high fevers, may require a doctor's attention. Make sure to stay fully hydrated. Your doctor may also prescribe an antibiotic. The diarrhea should end as your gut heals and your normal healthy population of gut bacteria is reestablished. I would not recommend using anti-diarrheal drugs such as loperamind, alosetron or diphenoxylate to treat diarrhea as these medications can have serious side effects.

Complex motility issues associated with diabetes (vagus nerve damage), hypothyroidism (hormonal and neuromuscular problems), scarring of the intestinal mucosal surface (Crohn's disease or scleroderma), surgery, and trauma should be discussed with your medical provider as these motility issues are outside the scope of this book.

Antibiotic Use

The problem with antibiotics is that they are indiscriminate bacteria killers. They certainly have valuable medical applications, but they can also disturb the balance of good to bad bacteria in the intestines — causing diarrhea and other problems. Whenever people take antibiotics, regardless of the reason, a large number of intestinal bacteria are killed. In most cases, the natural balance of your intestinal bacteria will be restored over time after you stop taking the antibiotic, but this can take a long time, even years. The biggest risk comes from broad-spectrum antibiotics, which kill a wide variety of bacteria. Ironically, these are the same drugs often used to treat SIBO-related disorders.

Broad-spectrum antibiotics can create an opportunity for toxic bacteria such as *C diff* to dominate the bacterial population. *C diff* overgrowth can cause a dangerous condition called pseudomembranous colitis (a serious inflammation of the large intestine). Even more powerful antibiotics may be required to treat this condition.

Antibiotic usage has been clearly linked to irritable bowel syndrome (IBS), which, in turn, has been linked to SIBO and GERD.

There are five reasons I am against using antibiotics for treating SIBO or any other condition except where there is a very clear medical need:

> *Antibiotics lack both short- and long-term efficacy for SIBO.*
>
> *Antibiotics kill both good and bad bacteria.*
>
> *Overusing antibiotics breeds resistant bacterial strains.*
>
> *Antibiotics are associated with side effects and can cause allergic reactions.*
>
> *There are better ways to control SIBO, particularly, in this case, the Fast Tract Diet.*

Symptoms such as abdominal pain, cramps, gas, bloating, diarrhea, reflux, etc. are indicative of SIBO, but if your symptoms come after you've taken a course of antibiotics, it's probably a good idea to talk to your health care provider. Your symptoms could indicate a more serious problem.

Treating Complications From Antibiotic Treatments

If possible, avoid antibiotics unless they are absolutely needed. This is the best way to avoid their complications and side effects.

Reestablishing the healthy balance of bacterial populations after taking antibiotics can take weeks, months, or in some cases, years. The Fast Tract approach can help you recover more quickly by limiting the amount of fermentable nutrients in your diet.

You may also try adding a high-quality probiotic supplement to your diet. High-quality probiotics typically contain live (freeze-dried) lactic acid bacteria such as *Lactobacillus acidophilis* and *Bifidobacteria*, usually containing over two billion cfu (colony forming units) per dose. In choosing a probiotic supplement make sure the following criteria are met:

> *The label should state the potency (how many bacteria per dose) and the expiration date. Probiotics manufactured in Canada are required to have an expiration date (supported by shelf life testing) but there is no identical requirement in the US.*

> *The probiotics should be shipped and stored under the recommended storage conditions.*

> *The probiotics should be protected with an enteric coating to ensure the bacteria survive their exposure to stomach acid.*

Instead of probiotics, some people consume a daily serving of yogurt that contains live gut-healthy bacteria including both *Lactobacillus acidophilis* and *Bifidobacteria*. One drawback of yogurt is that a large number of the bacteria will be killed by stomach acid.

Both probiotic supplements and yogurt contain only two or three different types of bacteria where the healthy gut contains hundreds of different species. So supplementing with two or three types may not provide a complete solution. If you decide to add daily yogurt to your diet, be sure to consult the tables in the appendix to select a type with limited fermentation potential.

Gastric (Stomach) Acid Reduction

Low stomach acid, called hypochlorhydria, is a common problem that puts people at a greater risk for developing SIBO, while increasing the difficulty of treating it. Without adequate stomach acid, bacteria eaten with food or liquids are no longer killed in the stomach. The stomach and upper intestine also become less acidic and more hospitable to the kind of bacterial growth that causes SIBO and GERD.

If you are taking PPI drugs to treat GERD or another condition, you don't need to be tested. You know that you have low stomach acid. That's what PPI drugs do.

I suggest you discuss the Fast Tract Diet with your doctor, and consider weaning yourself off PPIs that you're taking over a period of two to three weeks. Stopping PPI treatment without gradually decreasing your dosage can cause a potentially painful rebound effect.

Normally, the stomach plays a dual role: It both protects the intestines against outside threats from bacteria, viruses and parasites and protects the esophagus, lungs and sinuses from bacteria present in the digestive tract. Without stomach acid, this dual protection no longer exists. You'll not only be more susceptible to SIBO and related conditions, but also to pneumonia, asthma and sinus infections.

In this light, the well-documented connection between GERD and asthma makes perfect sense as does the connection between PPI drugs and pneumonia. Low acidity promotes SIBO, SIBO promotes gastroesophageal reflux, and reflux allows intestinal bacteria to enter the esophagus and lungs.

Several conditions can reduce or eliminate stomach acid. They include:

Most Common

Chronic use of acid-reducing medicines (antacids, H2 or PPI drugs). One study showed that as many as 50 percent of people taking PPI drugs suffered from bacterial overgrowth.[40]

Aging. As people get older, they often produce lower amounts of stomach acid, which is another reason (besides motility issues) why older people frequently suffer from SIBO-related illnesses including GERD.

H. Pylori infection. The bacterium that causes ulcers can reduce the amount of acid in the stomach. There is a test for H. pylori and the infection is treatable with antibiotics.

Less Common

Gastric bypass surgery.

Autoimmune disorders.

Stomach cancer. Stomach cancer can affect acid-producing parietal cells sharply reducing stomach acid production.

Radiation therapy. This is another way to damage acid-producing parietal cells.

Treating Reduced Stomach Acidity

Aging and the pervasive use of acid-reducing drugs are the most important factors. It's normal to lose the ability to produce the same quantity of stomach acid as you grow older. People over 50 with SIBO-related conditions can be tested, but finding doctors to perform the test might not be easy.

If testing shows you have low stomach acid (in the absence of an obvious cause), you might want to take betaine hydrochloride supplements (also known as betaine HCL) at the beginning of every meal. This will increase the overall level of stomach acid while you eat. Make sure not to take the supplements on an empty stomach.

Immune Impairment

The human immune system is made up of complex interactions between white blood cells, antibodies, proteins, cytokine-modulating factors and bile salts produced in the liver. Protective barriers such as your skin and your intestinal mucosal surface are considered to be part of your immune system. This complicated system protects us from viruses, bacteria, protozoa, and other pathogens and helps enforce order amongst the intestinal microflora.

A healthy immune system is critical to maintaining a balance of the type and number of bacteria present in the small intestine. Our immune system is able to tell the good bacteria from the bad (although the exact mechanism(s) are not clear). Though highly redundant, the system can be disturbed or damaged by a variety of factors. Cancer therapy, autoimmune conditions, the drugs to treat them, allergy and other medicines, HIV infection, illness and aging all can affect immunity.

Treating Immune Impairment

If possible, treating conditions that damage or disrupt your immune system will improve your ability to control SIBO. If you suspect you suffer from immune deficiencies, diagnostic testing is available that can help you determine what if any, immune impairments exist, and offer a path for treatment.

Many drugs can impair the immune system. The most common are drugs that treat autoimmune diseases and to some extent allergies, because autoimmune diseases and allergies are caused by an overactive or mis-directed immune system. Before making any changes to your medication, be sure to consult with your health care provider. It may be possible to change the type or dosage of any medication that's causing the problem.

Carbohydrate Malabsorption

In a general sense, malabsorption is the failure to absorb specific nutrients from the small intestine into the blood stream during digestion. Malabsorption can affect all three food groups — proteins, fats and carbohydrates — as well as vitamins and minerals. This can lead to a variety of illnesses, conditions, and nutritional deficiencies.[41]

Malabsorption has been referred to as the hallmark of SIBO. Not only does SIBO cause malabsorption, but malabsorption of carbohydrates is required for SIBO. Without malabsorbed carbohydrates, bacteria do not have the fuel required for overgrowth. In the next few chapters you'll see how this key concept provides the basis for the Fast Tract Diet.

Carbohydrates make up a significant portion of most people's diet. Many of these carbohydrates are difficult to digest, so carbohydrate malabsorption is common.

Carbohydrates range in size and complexity from small single-unit monosaccharides and double-unit disaccharides to very large polysaccharides linking together thousands of sugar units. Size is not always the determining factor in how easy carbohydrates are to break down and absorb. The molecular bonds holding the sugar units together also determine how digestible they are.

Many people have difficulty digesting and absorbing carbohydrate foods due to short-term illnesses, surgery or underlying chronic conditions.

Also, many carbohydrates are inherently difficult to digest and absorb even for people with fully functional digestive systems.

Carbohydrate malabsorption can be caused by the following:

> *Damage to the intestinal epithelium (from drugs, infections, SIBO or inflammation).*
> *Difficult-to-digest carbohydrates and sugar alcohols. These carbohydrates often escape digestion and absorption but are fermentable by intestinal bacteria.*
> *Overconsumption of carbohydrates, in general.*
>
> *Digestive enzyme deficiency (caused by pancreas problems, cystic fibrosis, or genetics).*

Damage to the Intestinal Epithelium

The interior surface of the intestine is lined with specialized epithelial cells that can be damaged by drugs (such as neomycin), SIBO, intestinal infections or inflammatory reactions. The key area of concern is the "brush border" area in the jejunum portion of the small intestine. Damage to this area destroys digestive enzymes and nutrient transport systems necessary for the final steps of digestion.

Several types of bacteria identified with SIBO, such as *Bacteroides fragilis*, *Clostridium perfringens*, and *Streptococcus fecalis*, possess protein-degrading enzymes that can destroy brush border enzymes including lactase, sucrase, and maltase, which are necessary for the final breakdown and absorption of carbohydrates.[42]

The ability of bacteria to damage critical digestive enzymes on the surface of the small intestine helps explain how SIBO causes carbohydrate malabsorption. Malabsorption of fats and fat-soluble vitamins may also be affected because many of the bacterial strains associated with SIBO can metabolize bile salts (needed for fat digestion).

Gastrointestinal infection, also known as gastroenteritis, is caused by bacteria such as *Salmonella, Shigella, Campylobacter, Cholera* and pathogenic *Escherichia coli*. Parasites such as *Giardia* or viruses can also cause gastroenteritis. Eating contaminated food, drinking or swimming in contaminated water or oral-fecal transmission is how most infections begin. Unlike SIBO, which is caused by an overgrowth of bacteria normally present in our intestines, gastroenteritis is typically caused by a single strain of disease-causing bacteria, parasite or virus that is not normally present in the digestive tract.

The symptoms of gastroenteritis tend to be sudden and dramatic, including stomach pain, vomiting, fever, and watery diarrhea. Most of the time the symptoms will resolve without treatment as the infection runs its course, but sometimes antibiotics or other drug treatments are required. The primary treatment is giving oral rehydration salts to replace water and electrolytes lost due to diarrhea. Gastroenteritis kills millions of people each year and is a leading cause of death in infants and young children. But gastroenteritis can also damage the intestinal epithelium, increasing carbohydrate malabsorption, and the likelihood of SIBO.

Autoimmune diseases such as celiac disease and Crohn's disease can also damage cells lining the small intestine. One study examined lactose malabsorption in Crohn's disease, an autoimmune disease characterized by intestinal inflammation. Crohn's disease patients showed a higher rate of lactose malabsorption.[43]

Treatment For Intestinal Surface Damage

There is no quick fix for damage to the surface of the small intestine. But the body has remarkable healing abilities. The important thing is to stop the cause of the damage, which can involve bacterial overgrowth, intestinal infection or food poisoning, or an autoimmune reaction from gluten (in the case of celiac disease). The small intestine can heal in one month or many months depending on the seriousness of the damage and the effectiveness of the treatment.

Volume-Based Carbohydrate Malabsorption

Early in the history of the human race every scrap of food was important. Calories were the key to our survival. Based on mutual survival needs humans evolved in partnership with microorganisms. By harboring a diverse population of microorganisms in our gut, we gained the ability to digest a wider variety of carbohydrates. These bacteria possessed unique enzymes that could help break down complex carbohydrates that our bodies could not digest. We were able to do this by adapting to use bacterial end products to help meet our own energy needs.

Fast forward to modern Western cultures. Today, we find ourselves surrounded by dietary excess. We can eat pretty much whatever we want whenever we want. The problem is that our survival instincts are like little voices telling us to eat as much as possible whenever we get a chance. In the paleolithic part of our brains, it may be the last meal we have for days. We all know "less is better," but our cravings and our instincts tempt us to overindulge. Deciding what foods to eat in what quantity and what foods to avoid can be challenging.

Too often, people indiscriminately overeat to the point where they suffer from a variety of serious health problems. In terms of digestive health threats, difficult to digest carbohydrates are the biggest problem, but volume-based malabsorption can also cause SIBO. Even though our body possesses very efficient digestive machinery, it can be overcome by sheer volume. I believe this is why obesity is linked to GERD and IBS[44] as well as symptoms such as bloating and diarrhea — hallmarks of malabsorption.[45]

Obesity often involves the consumption of large amounts of snack foods loaded with difficult-to-digest carbohydrates. Malabsorption is almost certain to occur, leading to conditions linked to SIBO, such as GERD and IBS.

Treating Difficult to Digest Carbohydrates

Finding ways to reduce the impact of difficult-to-digest carbohydrates is the main focus of this book, and the central design principle of the Fast Tract Diet. Almost every chapter in this book discusses ways you can improve the efficiency of your digestion!

Digestive Enzyme Deficiency

Finally, the disappearance of digestive enzymes as a result of pancreatic diseases, cystic fibrosis, lactose intolerance, or damage to the enzymes of the small intestine can also cause malabsorption and SIBO.

We know that digestive enzymes play a central role in the breakdown of fats, carbohydrates and proteins. Digestive enzymes are secreted with saliva in the mouth, produced and secreted by cells that line the stomach, and produced by the pancreas for secretion into the intestines. The cells that line the intestinal brush border produce still more digestive enzymes. While the loss of any digestive enzyme can contribute to nutrient malabsorption and digestive problems, the loss of carbohydrate-degrading enzymes (especially amylase, lactase and brush border enzymes) limit starch and sugar digestion and absorption providing the most powerful fuel for the development of SIBO.

Treating Digestive Enzyme Deficiency

The good news is that replacement enzymes can be taken as supplements to address two types of enzyme deficiencies — amylase and lactase deficiencies.

Enzyme replacement therapy may be appropriate for conditions such as lactose intolerance, cystic fibrosis, pancreatic cancer, and chronic pancreatitis. SIBO is common in these cases, because of the failure of the digestive enzymes and the malabsorption that follows.

Unless these enzymes are replaced with supplements, SIBO will be more difficult to treat and will require further dietary restriction. Without sufficient amylase, even amylopectin starch, allowed on the Fast Tract diet, can potentially cause symptoms.

If you believe you suffer from lactose intolerance or a condition resulting in amylase enzyme deficiency, talk to your health care provider. You may need to add a high-quality enteric-coated lactase or amylase enzyme supplement to your diet. Generally, you'll take one tablet or capsule before each meal. Be sure to check the expiration date, and store the supplements as directed on the label.

In the chapter that follows, our focus will turn from the organic issues that can put your digestive tract at risk of SIBO and GERD to the foods themselves. The typical diet consists of an extremely broad range of foods, some of which are easy to digest, and some of which are extremely difficult to digest. You can reduce your GERD symptoms by identifying and limiting your consumption of foods that will overwhelm your digestive system with undigested (and therefore fermentable) carbohydrates.

Chapter 7: Foods That Lead To SIBO

Now that you have a better idea of how underlying digestive issues can increase the likelihood of SIBO and GERD, I'd like to take a closer look at the critical dietary aspect of this problem — the foods that are more difficult to digest, and how they contribute to the problem.

A number of studies have shown that some carbohydrates are digested and absorbed better than others. The carbohydrates most subject to poor or incomplete absorption include:

Lactose

Fructose

Resistant starch

Fiber

Sugar alcohols (which are similar to carbohydrates)

While digestive health problems associated with lactose, fructose and even sugar alcohols have been widely documented, resistant starch and dietary fiber is widely considered to be healthy for the colon.

This is especially true for fiber, which is widely marketed in many forms as a key ingredient for digestive health. I was surprised to find little support for these claims in my research and now believe them to be exaggerated, dogmatic, and heavily promoted by companies that sell fiber-based products.

But the key issue for our purposes is that resistant starch and many types of fiber resemble lactose, fructose and sugar alcohols in their ability to persist in the intestine, providing a source of fermentable carbohydrates that can promote bacterial overgrowth.

For many people, the problem is simply over-consumption of these difficult-to-digest carbohydrates. But some individuals also have problems with digesting even small quantities of foods containing specific kinds of carbohydrates due to a variety of contributing factors. With that in mind, I'd like to give you a closer look at these prime "candidates" for malabsorption as well as the best available strategies for reducing their impact on your health.

Lactose

As discussed in chapter 2, lactose is a disaccharide (or double sugar) made of galactose and glucose that is present in milk, ice cream, cheese, and other dairy products made from milk.

Lactose intolerance and lactose malabsorption are essentially the same thing. Lactose intolerance is the inability to digest and absorb lactose. It's usually caused by a naturally occurring shortage or absence of the enzyme lactase, produced by the cells that line the small intestine. Lactase breaks down lactose into glucose and galactose that can then be absorbed into the bloodstream.

Most infants possess ample amounts of lactase, which helps them to digest and absorb the lactose in breast milk. For most people, lactase levels decrease with age after weaning. While most Northern Europeans are lactose-tolerant, the majority of people in many other parts of the world, such as Africa and Asia, are lactose-intolerant. Up to 50 million people in the US exhibit some level of lactose intolerance, and it affects approximately 75% to 80% of African and Asian Americans, and 90% of Native Americans (according to the National Institute of Diabetes and Digestive and Kidney Diseases (NIDDK)).

If your body does not produce enough lactase enzyme, you cannot digest lactose sugar or absorb it into your blood stream. The unabsorbed sugar is then fermented by bacteria in the small or large intestine. Lactose is an easy target for the bacteria in the small intestine and fully capable of fueling SIBO. The symptoms of lactose intolerance include nausea, cramps, bloating, diarrhea, gas and reflux following meals or snacks containing lactose.

If you experience symptoms of GERD (heartburn, etc.) or even IBS (cramps, diarrhea, etc.) after consuming milk or milk products, you may be lactose-intolerant and suffering from SIBO. If you see a doctor about these symptoms, he or she will most likely encourage you to avoid foods that contain lactose. If your symptoms improve after you remove lactose from your diet, you are almost certainly lactose-intolerant. Specific tests are available, but they are usually not necessary.

However, you may be affected by more than one cause (or contributing factor) of SIBO, and in this case it can be useful to have more specific testing done. Conditions that damage intestinal villi such as celiac or Crohn's disease can also lead to lactose malabsorption since the cells that produce the lactase enzyme have been damaged. Lactose intolerance caused by damaged villi can usually be reversed if treatment of the underlying cause, such as celiac or Crohn's disease, is effective.

Your health care provider can confirm lactose intolerance with a lactose tolerance test. After you drink a solution containing lactose, your blood glucose level is measured over a few hours to see how much lactose was converted to glucose and absorbed into your blood. If only a small amount of glucose enters the blood compared to the amount of lactose consumed, you will be diagnosed as lactose-intolerant. Hydrogen breath testing is another way to test for lactose malabsorption (refer to section on how to diagnose malabsorption and SIBO in chapter 6).

Treating Lactose Intolerance

Lactose intolerance can be treated in several different ways. One approach is to avoid milk and other lactose-containing foods, replacing them with lactose-free or reduced lactose products. A second approach is to take lactase enzyme supplements, which are available in both pill and liquid form, whenever you consume lactose-containing foods. This strategy can be very effective but requires diligence on your part.

Fortunately, most lactose-intolerant people still make some lactase and small amounts of lactose typically do not cause symptoms. Reducing the total amount of lactose you consume to less than 10 grams per day may be enough. If you fall into this category, you may be able to minimize your symptoms by avoiding milk that contains lactose (which has the highest level of lactose in common foods) while consuming moderate levels of other dairy products. You'll probably be best off with fermented dairy products such as cheese and yogurt where bacteria have already consumed most of the lactose during the fermentation process.

Yogurt, for example, contains lactase enzyme released by the bacteria while fermenting lactose. Studies have shown that the lactase in yogurt can make up for missing human lactase, making lactose digestion safe for most lactose-intolerant people when consumed with a yogurt "supplement."[46]

The Fast Tract Diet should solve the problem for most people. Dietary lactose increases fermentative potential, and lactose-containing foods are automatically limited with the Fast Tract Diet.

Fructose

Fructose is a monosaccharide (or single sugar) that requires no breakdown or digestion before it enters the bloodstream. Fructose intolerance and fructose malabsorption both refer to the body's inability to absorb fructose from the intestine into the blood stream.

Fructose malabsorption is common, affecting 39 to 50 percent of the population.[47] This condition is not related to hereditary fructose intolerance where the enzymes needed to breakdown fructose are simply missing. Hereditary fructose intolerance is a rare and serious condition beyond the scope of this book.

The symptoms of fructose malabsorption can include nausea, cramps, bloating, gas, reflux and diarrhea, which reflect the link between malabsorption, IBS, GERD and SIBO. As with lactose malabsorption, fructose malabsorption can be detected using a hydrogen breath test. In this case, fructose is given orally in place of lactose during the test.

Unlike glucose, which is absorbed directly into the blood stream as soon as it reaches the small intestine, fructose requires a much slower process, known as "facilitated diffusion," before it can be absorbed. Fructose connects with a protein called Glut 5 to pass through cells called enterocytes that line the intestine. You can compare glucose and fructose absorption to a daily commute to work via either a high-speed train (glucose) or riding a skateboard (fructose). Fructose has to "ride the skateboard" to go to work in the bloodstream.

Making the relatively slow and inefficient process even worse, people who have difficulty absorbing fructose may also be deficient in Glut 5, meaning that they, in effect, are trying to ride a broken skate board.[48]

Secondary causes of fructose malabsorption include damage to the intestinal surface caused by Crohn's disease, celiac disease, or SIBO itself.

Treating Fructose Intolerance

The most common treatment for fructose malabsorption is avoiding fructose and the related fructans. Fructans are categorized as fructo-oligosaccharides (chains of fructose containing less than ten fructose units), and inulins (chains of fructose containing more than 10 fructose units) and are actually more closely related to dietary fiber.

Unlike lactose intolerance, there is no supplement or enzyme that can help reduce fructose malabsorption. And avoiding fructose is a challenge because this sugar is present in so many foods and sweeteners. Fructose is the sweetener of choice in the food industry because it's much sweeter than glucose and other sugars. Even dietetic foods use fructose because less fructose is required to achieve the same sweetness.

Fructose makes up 50% of the sugar in sucrose and honey and just over half of the sugar in high fructose corn syrup. Glucose represents the balance of the sugar in these sweeteners. Other sweeteners containing fructose include maple syrup, molasses, and corn-based sweeteners. Fructose is also found in a wide variety of foods including candy, fruit, especially dried fruits such as raisins, figs and dates, fruit juices, soda, and vegetables.

Although research studies have not directly linked fructose to GERD, studies of IBS have shown that 85 percent of patients with IBS symptoms could reduce their impact by avoiding dietary fructose.[49] IBS and GERD are closely related, meaning that many people with IBS have GERD and many people with GERD have IBS. This demonstrated link between fructose malabsorption and IBS means that there's every reason to believe that avoiding fructose will help with GERD symptoms as well.

The exact mechanism isn't clear, but fructose absorption seems to improve dramatically in the presence of glucose. One study of 10 healthy volunteers showed evidence of fructose malabsorption with as little as 15 grams of fructose. When the same 10 subjects were given 100 grams of sucrose (a disaccharide made up of one unit of glucose and one unit of fructose), or 50 grams of fructose with 50 grams of glucose, there was no evidence of malabsorption.[50]

These results suggest that glucose stimulates or assists in the absorption of fructose. That's why sucrose, which is composed of equal amounts of fructose and glucose, is less likely to result in malabsorption than pure fructose. Similarly, high fructose corn syrup (HFCS), containing close to equal proportions of glucose and fructose, is less likely to cause malabsorption than pure fructose.

There is also evidence that fructose not only plays a role in digestive problems, but also in diabetes, heart disease, high cholesterol, high blood pressure and blocked arteries – all more good reasons to limit fructose. One approach to treating fructose intolerance is to make an exhaustive list of all the foods that are high in fructose — and avoid those foods. The alternative is to use the Fast Tract Diet, which makes it easy to limit all difficult-to-digest carbohydrates, including fructose.

Resistant Starch

Starch is a large complex carbohydrate used by plants such as oats, corn, potatoes, wheat, and rice to store energy. Foods that contain starch make up a large part of many people's diet.

For many years it was believed that starch was completely digested and absorbed in the small intestine. But studies published in the 1980s, based on hydrogen breath testing, showed that oats, wheat, potatoes, corn, and beans contained 10 to 20 percent malabsorbed, fermentable material.[51] In another study of the digestion of starch, samples were taken from the terminal ilium (the end of the small intestine) of healthy individuals after two different meals containing starch. This study showed that eight to 10 percent of the starch escaped absorption.[52] Even the digestion of bread, long known as the "staff of life," has been shown to end in malabsorption by hydrogen breath testing and symptom scoring.[53] Starch that isn't absorbed, known by scientists as "resistant starch," is estimated to represent at least 10 percent of the total starch in a typically Western diet. If ten percent of starch is malabsorbed in healthy people, how much is malabsorbed by people with digestive problems? The amount is certainly much higher.

Resistant starch is found in seeds, nuts, whole grains, cereals, bread, pasta, most rice varieties, most potato varieties, corn, certain fruits such as unripe bananas, and legumes such as beans and lentils. Undercooked, or cooked, then cooled foods contain more resistant starch than fully cooked or hot foods. In many ways, resistant starch is similar to and behaves like fermentable fiber in the digestive tract.

Resistant starch (RS) has been assigned to four groups based on the properties that allow it to resist digestion:[54]

> *RS1 - Physically resists digestion because of a protective matrix or coating surrounding the granules found in whole grains, legumes and seeds.*

> *RS2 – Is intrinsically resistant to digestion before cooking. RS2 includes unripe bananas, uncooked potatoes, along with many other foods.*

> *RS3 – Retrograded starch is formed when starchy foods are cooked and then cooled.*

> *RS4 – Refers to starch that is chemically modified to resist digestion and absorption. RS4 starches are often developed for use in processed foods.*

Several factors contribute to the formation of resistant starch, and, the relative amount of resistant starch in foods influences the level of malabsorption. The most important, yet often overlooked, factor is the ratio of the two molecular types of starch, amylose and amylopectin. Each type of starch possesses a unique structure and different properties that affect how easily they can be digested and absorbed.

Amylopectin, which is easy to digest and absorb, is a much larger molecule, containing 10,000 to 100,000 glucose units. At the molecular level amylopectin is highly branched. (See figure 17.) The large size and branching forms starch granules that are less dense and gelatinize (absorb water) easily when heated in water. Gelatinized starch is easier to digest. The branched, less dense structure also allows the digestive enzyme amylase to work more efficiently, breaking amylopectin down quickly into glucose, which is absorbed rapidly.

Amylose, which is more difficult to digest and absorb, is both smaller, containing only 100 to 10,000 glucose units, and less heavily branched compared to amylopectin. (Again, see figure 17.) This linear shape allows amylose to pack more tightly into the less accessible regions of starch granules where it's more difficult to digest.[55] A high ratio of amylose in starch granules also makes it more difficult to gelatinize (it gelatinizes at a higher temperature), making digestion by amylase even more difficult.

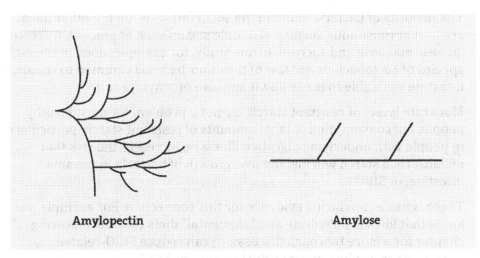

Amylopectin   **Amylose**

Figure 17. Branching nature of **amylopectin** *(highly branched)* and **amylose** *(fewer branches)* starch

Resistant starch (types RS1 through RS4) can contain both amylopectin and amylose. Comparing amylose content with glycemic index (how quickly foods are converted to blood sugar) reveals that amylose clearly represents the predominant component of resistant starch. In RS3, linear or straight portions of amylose can re-associate, forming insoluble crystallites that are difficult to digest.[56]

In general, foods that contain more amylopectin, such as jasmine rice, short grain and sushi rice as well as some varieties of potatoes, such as Russet Burbank, are much easier to digest and absorb than foods containing more amylose, such as basmati rice, most long grain rice (except for jasmine), pasta, most wheat, corn, oat and barley products, most potatoes and green bananas.

We know that a typical diet contains lots of resistant starch and we know that starch malabsorption is common. How does the presence of resistant starch affect the development of SIBO, and in turn GERD?

Resistant starch is fermentable by the bacteria common to the large intestine, including *Bifidobacterium, Clostridium, Bacteroides, Fusobacterium* and *Butyrivibrio*. These bacteria contain efficient starch-degrading enzymes and most can break down both amylopectin and amylose starch.[57]

The majority of bacteria found in the small intestine, on the other hand, are best at consuming single and double sugars such as glucose, fructose, lactose, mannose and sucrose. In one study, for example, none of the eight species of *Lactobacillus* and few of the other bacteria common to the small intestine were able to break down amylose or amylopectin.[58]

Moderate levels of resistant starch are not a problem for most healthy people, but consumption of large amounts of resistant starch, particularly in people with underlying digestive illnesses, increases the risk that malabsorbed starch will fuel the overgrowth of bacteria in the small intestine, or SIBO.

There is more convincing evidence for this connection. For example, we know that low-carbohydrate and "elemental" diets (see the following chapter for a more thorough discussion) can reduce SIBO-related intestinal gas production and GERD symptoms.[59]

As I mentioned earlier, there is also a strong link between cystic fibrosis and GERD. About 80% of cystic fibrosis patients suffer from GERD compared to about 20% in the general population. No one has been able to figure out exactly why. Cystic fibrosis patients, however, have a well-known deficiency of digestive enzymes, including a lack of pancreatic alpha amylase, an enzyme required for starch digestion. (The amylase present in saliva gets destroyed in the stomach.) The amylase cannot get out of the pancreas, where it's produced, because the pancreatic ducts are plugged up with thick mucus, a hallmark of CF.

Not surprisingly, this amylase deficiency results in starch malabsorption and SIBO. A study of CF patients with pancreatic deficiencies showed that SIBO was diagnosed (based on hydrogen breath testing) almost three times more frequently when compared to patients without cystic fibrosis.[60]

Surprisingly enough, there are actually products on the market that promote starch malabsorption. Weight loss products that block the absorption of starch are intentionally designed to inhibit amylase, the enzyme that normally breaks down starch. The idea behind these products is that blocking starch from being absorbed into the blood stream will prevent weight gain.

While the goal makes sense, the approach is short-sighted because it does not consider the possible consequences of malabsorption: diarrhea, cramps, bloating, abdominal distention, excessive gas and heartburn. Not so surprisingly, the side effects caused by these starch blockers include the symptoms of SIBO and GERD. The nearly inescapable conclusion is that starch malabsorption can cause SIBO, and ultimately GERD.

Amylose vs. Amylopectin Starch

There's one more critical aspect of this connection: I believe amylose (rather than amylopectin) starch to be the real culprit — because of its greater ability to resist digestion.

The key role of amylose malabsorption can be demonstrated by comparing the ability of different kinds of rice, containing different ratios of amylose and amylopectin, to raise blood sugar levels. Rice containing a higher ratio of amylose to amylopectin raises blood sugar less than rice containing amylopectin but no amylose.[61] A greater rise in blood sugar level indicates better digestion and absorption; a lesser rise in blood sugar level indicates malabsorption.

This difference is reflected in the glycemic index (again, more on this later), which determines the ability of carbohydrate-containing foods to raise blood sugar levels. Foods high in amylopectin, such as Asian short grain or glutinous rice, have a high glycemic index (98%) because they are digested and absorbed almost as efficiently as glucose — which has a glycemic index of 100%. Foods high in amylose, such as basmati rice, have a much lower glycemic index (58%), indicative of starch malabsorption.

According to researcher Peter Born, abdominal complaints (indicative of carbohydrate malabsorption and SIBO) affect 30% or more of Western populations, but only 10% of Asian populations.[62] Fewer symptoms in Asian populations could be due in part to Asian preferences for short grain rice over long grain rice and other starch containing foods. Short grain rice contains no amylose (only amylopectin) while most long grain rice varieties, such as basmati rice, and other starchy foods consumed by Western and other non-Asian cultures contain 20 to 30% amylose.

If you follow this evidence to its logical conclusion, it's clear that amylose starch is difficult to digest and absorb, but easy for bacteria associated with SIBO to metabolize. This can lead to severe gastrointestinal symptoms, including GERD. Any program with the goal of reducing the symptoms of SIBO and GERD will need to find some way to reduce the impact of amylose starch on digestion.

Unfortunately, there doesn't seem to be a specific medical test for amylose starch malabsorption. Technically, an amylose intolerance test could be given the same way a lactose or fructose intolerance test is given — by using high amylose starch in place of lactose or fructose — either by monitoring the rise in blood glucose (measuring the efficiency of digestion and absorption) or by using a hydrogen breath test (measuring how much bacterial fermentation is occurring in the small intestine). The lack of such a test is probably due to the general lack of recognition of the role of amylose starch in carbohydrate malabsorption.

Treating Amylose Malabsorption

Because amylose starch is present in so many starchy vegetables, desserts, sauces, and baked goods, it would be difficult to avoid it completely. The best approach is to reduce how much amylose starch you consume by following a carefully designed eating plan, like the Fast Tract Diet. The Fast Tract Diet works by limiting all difficult to digest carbohydrates, including resistant (mostly amylose) starch.

Fiber

Fiber is the indigestible part of plant-based foods, consisting of structural components such as the cell walls of fruits, vegetables, nuts and legumes, the tough outer layers of grains, as well as any other non-digestible carbohydrates, as well as lignin — a substance found in plants that binds the cellulose fibers together. The quick list of dietary fibers includes:

Fructans (including inulin and other polymers of fructose)

Pectin

Beta glucan (polydextrose)

Gums

Stachyose

Raffinose

Verbascose

Hemicellulose

Cellulose

Lignin

Resistant starch (which we've just looked at in detail) is sometimes categorized as a type of dietary fiber because it exhibits similar properties, particularly in terms of indigestibility and fermentability. Similarly, sugar alcohols (mannitol, sorbitol, xylitol, erythritol, etc.) are not classified as fiber, yet like fiber, resist digestion and are fermentable by gut bacteria.

Soluble and Insoluble Fiber

Most plants contain both soluble and insoluble fiber. Soluble fiber includes pectin, polydextrose, some hemicelluloses, raffinose, stachyose, verbascose and fructans. Soluble fiber increases the viscosity of semi-solid materials moving through the intestines, increasing the time it takes to travel the entire route.

Insoluble fiber includes cellulose (beta-glucan), lignin and some hemicelluloses. Insoluble fiber is believed to increase bulk, soften stools and decrease gut transit time, potentially helping relieve constipation.

Because both soluble and insoluble fiber increases stool bulk, fiber can make you feel fuller. This has been proposed as an explanation of why fiber might help with weight loss.

Fiber Intake and Health

The Academy of Nutrition and Dietetics (AND) recommends consuming between 20 and 35 grams of fiber per day. Most people consume 14 grams per day or less.

It's proven to be extremely difficult to confirm the many reported health benefits of fiber in the diet. Companies that market foods that contain fiber certainly publicize these reported benefits, but supporting evidence is hard to find.

For example, in a clinical study looking at the use of bran to reduce constipation, 20 grams of bran per day did not improve constipation symptoms compared to the placebo.[63]

Fiber is also, by reputation, an important tool in lowering cholesterol. In the eighties, for instance, a small study reported that 60 grams of oat bran or oat meal per day lowered cholesterol levels by roughly 3% after 12 weeks — when combined with a low fat diet.[64] However, another study found that fiber had no cholesterol-lowering effect in men with high cholesterol who did not follow a low-fat diet.[65] A third study, at Brigham and Women's Hospital in Boston, Massachusetts, found that oat bran and low-fiber wheat had the same moderate effect on cholesterol levels, suggesting that fiber itself is not responsible.[66]

What about fiber and heart health? Two studies, one based in Finland and one in Japan suggest that people who eat lots of fiber (30-35 grams per day) may reduce their risk of coronary heart disease.[67]

I asked Gary Taubes, the author of *Good Calories Bad Calories*, about these studies. Gary cautioned me about reading too much into them. Observational studies follow large groups of people (22,000 subjects in the Finnish case, and 58,000 in the Japanese study) over time to see how their health develops. Then they compare, for example, the subgroup who ate the most fiber with the subgroup that ate the least, measure the occurrence of disease in each, and then draw conclusions about cause and effect connections.

He pointed out that the problem with this kind of study is that fiber consumption may not be the only factor shared by members of the subgroups. For example, the subgroup that ate more fiber may also be more health-conscious in general, and a more careful look at them might reveal that they also drink less, or smoke less, or exercise more. If true, this means that you cannot make a cause-and-effect connection between

72

fiber consumption and heart health based on these studies. (At least not without a lot more information about the individuals.)

For more information on the effect of biases on observational studies, you might be interested in a cover story Gary wrote for *The New York Times Magazine* in September 2007 entitled, "Do We Really Know What Makes Us Healthy?" Gary's point is that many hypotheses generated by observational studies later turn out not to be true, and setting broad dietary guidelines without randomized, placebo-controlled clinical studies can lead to unintended and sometimes unhealthy consequences.

Another example: The idea that high dietary fiber may lower the risk of colon cancer came from studies in the 1970s that made a connection between low colon cancer rates in developing countries and diets higher in fiber.[68] A more recent study of 88,757 women found no association between dietary fiber consumption and the risk for colon cancer.[69] Similar results were obtained from the Fukuoka Colorectal Cancer Study,[70] and another large study of men.[71]

I have to admit that these results surprised me. Like most people, I grew up believing in the health benefits of fiber. If fiber did no harm it might not matter. But unfortunately, that's not the case for many people with digestive problems. For these people, excessive dietary fiber can create significant health challenges, because it can lead to excessive intestinal fermentation, SIBO, and GERD.

For one thing, it's nearly impossible for most people to consume enough fiber on a daily basis to realize any potential health benefits.

And commercial fiber supplements often contain large amounts of added sugar, which can increase the potential for fermentation in the small intestine. For instance, the recommended dose of the fiber supplement Metamucil, which contains fiber from psyllium husk, is one tablespoon three times per day. This daily dose equals 9 grams of dietary (insoluble) fiber, 7 grams of soluble fiber, and 21 (!) grams of sugar.

By definition, the fiber in our diet is not digested or absorbed. The fiber we consume resists absorption and must pass through both the small and large intestine. Along the way, fiber is subjected to fermentation as a wide variety of bacteria try to break it down for energy.

Most fiber fermentation occurs in the large intestine and is generally considered normal and healthy. But consuming too much fiber can also cause excess fermentation in the small intestine. This can lead to serious gastrointestinal problems. Excessive fermentation in the small intestine increases the presence of bacterial endo- and exo- toxins as well as hydrogen, carbon dioxide, and methane gas. Symptoms can include pain, bloating, distention, gas, reflux, cramps, and diarrhea (and is some cases, constipation, especially in the absence of sufficient water).

Fermentability of Fiber Types

The "fermentability" of fiber depends on the chemical makeup of the fiber, as well as the amount and types of bacteria present in the small and large intestines. Bacteria normally present in the small intestine can ferment smaller disaccharide sugars along with some easier-to-digest types of fiber. Bacteria normally present in the large intestine use a range of enzymes to ferment even the most resistant fiber types.

Fructans are long chains of fructose that include fructooligosaccharide and inulin. They are found in wheat, artichokes, garlic, onions, unripe bananas, asparagus and green beans. Fructans are highly fermentable by some bacteria, notably *Bifidobacteria*, which is considered to be a healthy inhabitant of the large intestine but is also associated with SIBO. It has been suggested that fructans can promote intestinal health, but there is also solid evidence linking fructans to SIBO. One study, for instance, found that fructans cause abdominal symptoms that can be reversed by limiting their consumption.[72]

Pectin, on the other hand, tends to be metabolized slowly. In one study it took up to six hours to detect metabolic end products that indicated that gut bacteria in the large intestine had consumed the pectin.

Beta-glucan, present in oat flour, has been found to be highly fermentable resulting in gases as an end product.[73] Acacia gums used as food additives are also rapidly fermented by intestinal bacteria.[74]

Raffinose (trisaccharide), stachyose (tetrasaccharide) and verbascose (pentasaccharide) are found in legumes, especially beans, cabbage and Brussels sprouts. These fibers are well known for their role in causing flatulence, indicating that they are fermented in the large intestine. They are broken down by bacteria that possess the enzyme alpha-galactosidase (also present in the digestive supplement Beano). There is a risk that the excess gas produced by these fiber types could work its way into the small intestine and cause SIBO, or into the stomach and cause reflux.

In a study of fiber fermentability, cellulose was compared to water-insoluble hemicellulose and lignin.[75] The results show that 80 percent of the cellulose was fermented, with up to 15 percent of the fermentation taking place in the small intestine. Over 95 percent of the water-insoluble hemicellulose was fermented with up to 72 percent of the fermentation taking place in the small intestine. Lignin was not fermented at all.

Table 1. Relative Fermentability of Fiber Types.

Fiber Type	Fermentability
Beta glucans	High
Fructans	High
Gums	High
Stachyose	Medium
Raffinose	Medium
Verbascos	Medium
Hemicellulose	Variable
Pectin	Low (safer form of fiber)
Cellulose	Low (safer form of fiber)
Lignin	Low (safer form of fiber)

Fiber, IBS and GERD

For decades, fiber was widely recommended as a treatment for Irritable Bowel Syndrome (IBS). But a study of wheat bran for IBS symptoms was inconclusive.[76] Along the same lines, treating 275 IBS patients with psyllium or bran fiber for three months did not improve their quality of life. The bran group actually suffered a high dropout rate because the participant's symptoms, including heartburn, kept getting worse.[77]

On the other hand, IBS patients who eliminated fiber from their diet showed a significant improvement in symptoms as well reduced production of hydrogen.[78] Avoiding fiber was actually more effective at reducing hydrogen gas than the potent antibiotic metronidazole. Since IBS, SIBO, and GERD are closely related, this research has important implication for people with GERD-related symptoms.

Treating Fiber Malabsorption

There's no real point in testing for fiber malabsorption since fiber, by definition, is not supposed to be digested or absorbed. But if excessive fiber causes excessive fermentation, a lactulose breath test should be able to detect possible SIBO.

Moreover, trying to limit types of fiber in the diet is difficult. There are so many different kinds that it is difficult to link symptoms with any specific type of fiber.

My advice would be to enjoy plenty of green, leafy, and stalked vegetables as well as nuts and seeds that contain the less fermentable types of fiber. But consume beans, lentils and legumes in limited quantities. Soy beans are easier to digest even though they have plenty of fiber, because they are lower in fermentable fiber and other carbohydrates.

Sugar Alcohols

Sugar alcohols, sometimes referred to as polyols, include sorbitol, mannitol, xylitol, lactitol, isomalt, erythritol, and maltitol. Sugar alcohols taste sweet, but are poorly digested and absorbed. One benefit is that they don't raise blood sugar as much or have as many calories as sugar. For this reason, sugar alcohols have been used for weight and diabetic control and for preventing dental cavities. Sugar alcohols are generally accepted as sugar-free alternatives for people on low carb diets.

While several sugar alcohols including xylitol, mannitol and sorbitol, are listed as GRAS (Generally Regarded As Safe) food additives by the FDA, not all sugar alcohols are included. The FDA requires that mannitol and sorbitol have warning labels indicating that over 20 grams per day for mannitol and 50 g per day for sorbitol can give a laxative effect. But these warnings don't appear to go far enough. For instance, early studies on sorbitol using hydrogen breath testing indicate that bacterial fermentation was observed with as little as 5 grams, and that at 10 grams, subjects experienced gas and bloating. The symptoms became more severe, including cramps and diarrhea, when 20 grams were ingested.[79] In another study, 84 percent of people ingesting 25 grams of sorbitol had a positive breath test for malabsorption and 57 percent exhibiting malabsorption reported symptoms.[80] Clearly people experience GI symptoms well below the 50 grams per day deemed by the FDA as acceptable.

While sugar alcohols have not been definitively linked to heartburn symptoms, the fact that these sweeteners cause bloating, cramps and diarrhea as well as excessive fermentation suggests that any diet for

GERD, a condition that is often linked to other GI symptoms, should limit these sweeteners.

Avoiding sugar alcohols can be hard to do as they are often added to cough syrup, mouthwash, toothpaste, baked goods, syrups, candy, gum, chocolate and other "sugarless" or diet products. To determine if products you buy contain sugar alcohols, check the labels. Luckily, the FDA requires food labels to list the amount (if not the specific types) of sugar alcohols. The Fast Tract Diet includes sugar alcohols when calculating fermentation potential and does not use or include sugar alcohols in the Fast Tract Diet recipes.

All of this information about food types is designed to prepare you for the next chapter in this book, where we take a quick look at some of diets that have been developed to treat digestive tract conditions. All of these diets try to limit foods that cause gastric distress, and increase your consumption of foods that do not.

Understanding the nature of the foods that your body is trying to digest will both help you understand why many diets do not fully protect your gastrointestinal tract from SIBO and GERD, and show you how the Fast Tract Diet that I've developed offers a safe, thorough and complete solution to the problem.

Chapter 8: Reducing The Risk In Your Diet

My research has established that SIBO and related digestive conditions such as GERD have many underlying causes, but the driving force behind SIBO is *always* poorly absorbed carbohydrates. The best way to limit SIBO — and GERD — is to deny gut bacteria the fuel they need to overrun the small intestine by limiting the consumption of hard-to-digest carbohydrates.

Several existing diets have shown promise in treating SIBO-related conditions. These include the Elemental Diet, Specific Carbohydrate Diet, Low Starch Diet, Low Carb Diet and the FODMAP approach. These diets all limit carbohydrate malabsorption; an approach known to be effective for treating SIBO. Unfortunately, none of them offers a completely effective treatment for SIBO or GERD.

The Elemental Diet

The Elemental diet consists of foods that are essentially "predigested." The foods contain fatty acids rather than fats, amino acids rather than proteins, and glucose instead of carbohydrates. The diet formula also includes water and micronutrients — vitamins and minerals. Elemental diet product such as Nestle's Vivonex can be delivered orally or enterally (by tube). Elemental diets are designed to ensure full absorption and have been used to treat a broad range of digestive conditions including: Crohn's and celiac disease, lactose intolerance, malabsorption, diarrhea, constipation, diabetes, cystic fibrosis, abdominal distention, and short bowel syndrome. Note that all of these conditions have some connection to SIBO. Some of the drawbacks of the elemental diet approach include high cost, unappealing (predigested!) food products, and the need for medical supervision.

The Specific Carbohydrate Diet

The book *Breaking the Vicious Cycle* by Elaine Gottschall describes her experiences with Drs. Sidney and Merrill Haas, who successfully treated celiac disease (linked to SIBO) with a diet that allowed only specific sugars and starches. The Specific Carbohydrate Diet limits disaccharide or double sugars as well as grains and starch, but allows simple sugars like glucose.

In general, this dietary approach is on the right track, but it fails to limit a number of known contributors to SIBO and GERD. For example, honey is used extensively in the recipes even though honey has just as much fructose as table sugar (sucrose is made of equal parts glucose and fructose). And the diet also allows a large variety of fruits and fruit juices that contain large quantities of fructose, which is now recognized as a major contributor to the development of SIBO.

Finally, the SCD does not allow any grains or foods containing starch. It wrongly identifies amylose starch as easy to digest and amylopectin starch as difficult to digest, suggesting that amylopectin and not amylose is more likely to cause microbial fermentation. The reverse is actually true.

Note: The GAPS Diet (Gut and Psychology Syndrome) created by Dr. Natasha Campbell-McBride is based on the Specific Carbohydrate Diet but also includes detoxification, and supplementation.

The Low Starch Diet

Carol Sinclair popularized the Low Starch Diet in her book *The IBS Low-Starch Diet*. Sinclair discovered that reducing starch in her diet improved her IBS symptoms. She also collaborated with Dr. Alan Ebringer, a professor of immunology at Kings College in London, UK, who found that the diet could improve painful symptoms of ankylosing spondylitis (AS). Dr. Ebringer has made the connection between the autoimmune disease AS, intestinal overgrowth of the bacterium *Klebsiella pneumonia*, and controlling the bacteria's growth through a low-starch diet. Sinclair's book limits all starches as well as sucrose, lactose and maltose.

Unfortunately, like the Specific Carbohydrate Diet, the Low Starch Diet does not limit fructose, and will not be completely effective in treating SIBO or GERD.

The Low Carb Diet

Dr. Robert Atkins made low carbohydrate dieting famous when he published *Diet Revolution* in the 1970s. Two other ground-breaking books on low-carb dieting; *Protein Power* by Drs. Mike and Mary Dan Eades and *Good Calories Bad Calories* by Gary Taube, show how low-carb dieting works at the biochemical level to improve human health beyond weight loss.

Studies have shown that strict (ketogenic) low-carb dieting can also improve IBS and GERD symptoms, two conditions associated with SIBO.[81] Despite impressive results (as documented in my first book, *Heartburn Cured*), not everyone with GERD gets complete symptom relief from a low carb diet. One possible explanation for the variations in results is that the low-carb diets don't restrict fiber — another well-known contributor to digestive illness. Another reason might be a simple failure to stick with the diet. Many people are unwilling to follow a strict low-carb eating plan for extended periods of time.

The FODMAP Approach

Susan Shepherd and Peter Gibson developed the FODMAP diet at Monash University in Victoria, Australia.[82] The acronym FODMAP represents four classes of fermentable sugars/sugar alcohols: Fermentable Oligo-, Di-, and Monosaccharides, And Polyols.[83] The FODMAP approach limits fructose, fructans, lactose, galactans and sugar alcohols.

One major flaw in the FODMAP approach is that it fails to limit resistant starch, a significant contributor to malabsorption and excessive fermentation. In fact, the FODMAP diet calls for adding more resistant starch. As a recent article on the diet stated, "Part of dietary counseling is to ensure continuing adequate intake of resistant starch."[84] Another drawback of the FODMAP system is that a trained dietitian must deliver it.[85]

The Fast Tract Diet

Fortunately, my research on the biochemistry of digestion points to a new way of understanding the connection between poor absorption, SIBO, and GERD. It has also led me to develop a "new kind of diet" that offers a safe, thorough, and easy to understand way to control malabsorption through avoiding certain foods.

The defining feature of the Fast Tract Diet is the method it uses to calculate the potential for any food containing carbohydrates to cause symptoms characteristic of SIBO and GERD. Mathematically derived values for the fermentation potential (FP) of different foods helps identify and restrict difficult-to-digest carbohydrates, notably fructose, lactose, fiber, amylose and sugar alcohol. None of the other diets limit the full list of difficult-to-digest carbohydrates that can promote SIBO. (The Specific and Low-Starch diets don't restrict fructose, the Low-Carb diets don't restrict sugar alcohols or fiber, and the FODMAP approach doesn't limit resistant starch.)

And, unlike the Elemental and FODMAP diets that require delivery by a medical professional or dietitian, anyone who reads this book can reduce their symptoms by following the recipes in Appendix B, or by creating their own recipes for foods with low FP values. I've done the hard work

81

for you — by calculating the fermentation potential of a broad range of common foods, and by combining low-FP foods in recipes and meal plans to ensure efficient and complete digestion and absorption.

The diet is based on balanced, nutritious and appetizing meals made with wholesome foods right off the grocery shelves.

Low-FP foods include low-amylose rice and potatoes, cheese, meats, tofu, some simple sugars (but not lactose and fructose), nuts, watermelon, berries, some types of bread, crackers, eggs, cream, lactose-free milk, dry wines, light beer, and non-starch vegetables.

Unlike purely low-carb diets, Fast Tract meals can include both low-carb foods and higher-carb foods as long as they don't contain too many difficult-to-digest carbohydrates.

Together, this leaves fewer carbs for gut microorganisms to consume. The result is less gas, less gas pressure and less reflux.

In a nutshell, the Fast Tract Diet represents a safe, effective, and flexible system to control SIBO, which I believe to be the real cause of GERD.

The next three chapters will give you a more complete introduction to the Fast Tract Diet. The first will explain how to calculate the fermentation potential of any given food, and how to use that information. The second presents a complete diet program — full of helpful tips and advice on how to get the most out of the Fast Tract Diet. Finally, the third chapter that follows offers scores of recipes and meal plans designed to help you control SIBO and GERD. That final chapter proves that you can eat well and be healthy without symptoms, even if you've been affected by GERD.

Chapter 9: Measuring Heartburn Risk in Foods

Soon after publishing my first book on GERD, I was fortunate enough to become friends with Dr. Mike Eades. I had asked Mike to review my book because he and his wife, Dr. Mary Dan Eades, had written about the benefits of low-carbohydrate diets for people affected by GERD in their bestselling book, *Protein Power*. Mike was intrigued by my theory that GERD is related to the poor absorption of carbohydrates and bacterial overgrowth. He asked me the following key question:

"Do all carbs trigger acid reflux and, if not, can you devise something like a barometer for heartburn that helps people avoid the worst carbs?"

I have spent the last three years answering that question. My insight was that the more difficult the carbohydrates were to digest, the more likely it was that some of the carbohydrates would not be digested or absorbed, and could serve as a source of food or fuel for gut bacteria. The higher the amount of malabsorption, the higher the rate of fermentation and production of gas in the digestive tract.

It turns out that avoiding five difficult to digest carbohydrates is the key to symptom relief. As I mentioned in previous chapters, they are fructose, lactose, resistant starch, fiber, and sugar alcohol (which is similar to a carbohydrate). But avoiding these five carbohydrates can be quite complex without a thorough knowledge of their types and amounts in all the foods you consume.

To overcome this burden, I needed to address the second part of Mike's question, and create a way to measure the total amount of difficult-to-digest carbohydrates in each food that would be subject to malabsorption and fermentation by gut bacteria.

The FP (Fermentation Potential) Breakthrough

It finally dawned on me that the glycemic index developed by Dr. David Jenkins at the University of Toronto could be used for this purpose. The GI measures the relative ease with which carbohydrates are digested and absorbed into the bloodstream, so it made sense that it could also be used to calculate the carbohydrates that are left over — not digested and absorbed into the bloodstream. I used the glycemic index and nutritional information (serving size, net carbs, fiber and sugar alcohol) for individual foods to calculate what I call the Fermentation Potential or FP.

If you know the serving size, total amount of net carbs (NC), dietary fiber (DF) and sugar alcohols (SA), and the glycemic index (GI) for a food, you can easily calculate the fermentation potential. For people suffering from SIBO-related symptoms such as acid reflux, the FP value is a systematic way to rate "symptom potential." Foods having a low FP will be much less likely to trigger symptoms than foods having a high FP.

The formula for FP looks like this:

$$FP = \frac{(100 - GI)xNC}{100} + DF + SA$$

The glycemic index of foods is based on the type of carbohydrates each food contains (sugars, starches, or fiber), how the food has been cooked or processed, the presence (or absence) of other foods, and how fast the food is eaten. The Glycemic Load (GL) measures the overall amount of carbohydrates expected to be absorbed into the blood stream for a typical serving of the food in question.

The only way to establish the glycemic index for a particular food is to test it in people.

Typically, individuals are tested in the morning, after an overnight fast. For the first three trials, they give a baseline blood sample, and then consume 50 grams of pure glucose. The concentration of glucose in their blood is measured in additional blood samples taken at 15, 30, 45, 60, 90 and 120 minutes after the baseline sample.

Whole blood glucose levels are measured with an automatic analyzer that can accurately determine the concentration of glucose in the blood. Measuring blood glucose levels over time (producing what's known as the "blood glucose response curve") gives a much more accurate value for glucose absorption than measuring blood glucose at a single point in time.

After the three trials with glucose, known as the reference food, the individuals are tested again, this time after consuming the food being studied. These results are then compared to the trials using glucose.

Glucose doesn't need to be digested or "broken down" — it is absorbed completely and directly into the blood stream. Pure glucose is absorbed so efficiently that you can expect 100 % of a 50-gram test dose to be absorbed into the blood stream. As a result, glucose is assigned a glycemic index of 100.

The glycemic index for a specific food can then be calculated by comparing its absorption to the absorption of pure glucose. The absorption value for 50 grams of the test food is divided by the absorption for 50 grams of glucose, and then multiplied by 100 to arrive at a glycemic index.

Here's the general equation:

GI (Glycemic Index)

= (absorption of 50 g test food) / absorption of 50 g glucose)
x (100)

Let's look at a simple example by calculating the glycemic index of spaghetti. While spaghetti's glycemic index varies depending on the type of spaghetti and how long it's cooked, the absorption value for a 180 gram (6.35 ounce) serving containing 50-grams of net carbs is typically around 22 grams.

According to our formula:

GI (glycemic index) = (22)/(50) x 100 = 44

In this case, the glycemic index of spaghetti was calculated to be 44. In other words, spaghetti raised blood sugar only 44% as much as pure glucose. That means that 44% of the 50-gram serving of spaghetti, or 22 grams (0.44 x 50g = 22 g), was absorbed into the blood stream. This amount is known as the Glycemic Load (GL).

This whole process is repeated for each new food tested. Since 1980, over 1000 carbohydrate-containing foods have been tested in this fashion. (The next time you see the glycemic index listed for an individual food, remember that a determined test subject was stuck with a needle 28 times to determine that number!)

The availability of good glycemic index data for many of the most common foods containing carbohydrates makes it possible to calculate the fermentation potential of these foods. If you know the total carbohydrates (including net carbohydrates, fiber, and sugar alcohol) of a food, and you know its glycemic index (measuring how much of it will be digested and absorbed), you can easily calculate the carbohydrates that will be "left over" to fuel fermentation.

The key question here is: "What happens to the carbohydrates that aren't absorbed?" To continue with our example, the question becomes, "if 44% of the carbohydrates in spaghetti are absorbed, what happens to the 56% (or 0.56 x 50 grams = 28 grams) that is not absorbed?" If 22 grams of carbohydrates from of a 50-gram serving of spaghetti enter the blood stream, the remaining 28 grams must remain in the intestines. And what about the fiber? A serving of pasta with 50 grams of carbohydrates contains about 3 grams of fiber. Fiber is a non-digested carbohydrate that needs to be included in the calculation.

Adding the 28 grams of net carbohydrate and the 3 grams of fiber from spaghetti gives us a total of 31 grams of carbohydrate left in the digestive tract after a meal — and available to be "fermented" by intestinal bacteria. Hopefully, most of this fermentation will take place in the large intestine, where fermentation is relatively normal, but the more "fuel" is left behind, the more likely it is that some of the fermentation will take place in the small intestine, raising the chances for SIBO to develop.

(Note that the serving size used in the FP tables for spaghetti is slightly less than the serving depicted in this example, and the FP value for the smaller serving will therefore be less than 31g.)

I refer to these unabsorbed carbohydrates as having "Fermentative Potential." The unabsorbed carbohydrates represent potential food for intestinal microorganisms. And remember that as little as 30 grams of malabsorbed carbohydrates (30 FP grams) can produce 10 liters of intestinal gas. That is a huge amount of gas. Imagine ten balloons filled with one liter of gas each. Then imagine these balloons inside your intestines!

Someone eating a typical American diet (for example — oatmeal, bread, and orange juice for breakfast; a banana for a snack; cheeseburger, fries and a soda for lunch; and rice, carrots, chicken, milk and chocolate cake for dinner) easily consumes a daily FP of more than 160 grams. That is the equivalent of more than 50 balloons per day!

The FP value, measuring unabsorbed carbohydrates, is much more valuable for people with GERD or other conditions caused by SIBO than either glycemic index (GI) or glycemic load (GL). Carbs with a low FP will be much less likely to cause acid reflux. The most heartburn friendly carb is glucose, which has a glycemic index of 100 (or 100%), it has a fermentation potential of zero, because it is completely absorbed into the bloodstream.

Finally, let's take a look at a few more sample calculations for common foods to see how to determine whether a given food is safe for you. These calculations are based on round numbers so that the calculation is easier to follow. For exact values, see the FP tables in Appendix C.

Bread Comparison

English Muffin (FP 4 g) — *Less Potential for Heartburn*
Serving size = 1 oz, 30 g
NC 14 g
Fiber 1 g
GI 77
FP = ((100 – 77) x 14)/100 + 1 = 4 g

Whole Grain Bread (FP 8g) — *More Potential for Heartburn*
Serving size = 1 oz, 30 g
NC 13 g
Fiber 2 g
GI 51
FP = ((100 – 51) x 13)/100 + 2 = 8 g

Comparing two types of bread products, you can see that FP can vary quite a bit. Keep in mind that many people with diagnosed and undiagnosed celiac disease can't tolerate the gluten in wheat products. Remember to chew bread and other starchy foods well before swallowing to give the amylase in your saliva ample time to breakdown the starch.

Yogurt Comparison

Plain Yogurt (FP 7 g) — *Less Potential for Heartburn*
Serving size 8 oz, 228 g
NC 10 g
Fiber 0 g
GI 36
FP = ((100 – 36) x 10) / 100 + 0 = 7 g

Sweetened Yogurt with Fruit (FP 23g) — *More Potential for Heartburn*
Serving size 8 oz, 228 g
NC 35 g

Fiber 0 g
GI 33
FP = ((100 – 33) x 35) / 100 + 0 = 23

Notice the difference between sweetened and unsweetened yogurt. The sweetened yogurt contains 16 more grams of difficult to digest carbs per serving. I recommend plain yogurt sweetened with Splenda or other non-sugar substitutes besides sugar alcohols.

Rice Comparison

Asian Sticky Rice (FP 3g) — *Less Potential for Heartburn*
Serving size 5.3 oz, 150 g
NC 32   g
Fiber 2 g
GI 98
FP = ((100 – 98) x 32) / 100 + 2 = 3 g

Jasmine Rice (FP - 4 g) — *Less Potential for Heartburn*
Serving size 5.3 oz, 150 g
NC 42 g
Fiber 0 g
GI 109
FP = ((100 – 109) x 42) / 100 + 0 = - 4 g

Basmati Rice (FP 17g) — *More Potential for Heartburn*
Serving size 5.3 oz, 150 g
NC 38 g
Fiber 1
GI 58
FP = ((100 – 58) x 38) / 100 + 1 = 17 g

Uncle Ben's White Rice (FP 20g) — *More Potential for Heartburn*
Serving size 5.3 oz, 150 g
NC 36 g
Fiber 0 g
GI 45
FP = ((100 – 45) x 36) / 100 + 0 = 20 g

In this comparison of rice varieties, you can see that Asian sticky rice (also known as glutinous rice) and jasmine rice have very low fermentation potentials indicating they are heartburn friendly. Jasmine rice has a negative FP indicating that it is actually absorbed faster than pure glucose due to its lack of amylose starch and perhaps the fluffy nature of its amylopectin starch content. Practically speaking, you can assume that 100% of the carbs in jasmine rice are absorbed and zero grams remain in the intestine. Asian sticky rice fairs almost as well with 97 grams absorbed and only 3 grams remaining in the intestine. Just remember not to over-consume any starch-containing food, eat slowly and chew well.

Other rice varieties don't fare as well in comparison. Basmati rice and Uncle Ben's white converted rice have FP values of 17 and 20 grams respectively. Every time you consume a serving of these rice varieties between 17 and 20 grams of difficult to digest carbs become available for gut fermentation. While this might be fine for people without intestinal bacterial overgrowth, it can be a problem for people with GERD and other related conditions. For this reason, the recipes in this book use only Asian short grain sticky rice and jasmine rice.

Pasta Comparison

Pasta (rice-based) (FP 5g) — *Less Potential for Heartburn:*
Serving size 6 oz, 170 g
NC 36 g
Fiber 2 g
GI 92
FP = ((100 – 92) x 36) / 100 + 2 = 5g

Pasta (wheat-based) (FP 28g) — *More Potential for Heartburn:*
Serving size 6 oz, 170 g
NC 45 g
Fiber 3 g
GI 44
FP = ((100 – 44) x 45) / 100 + 3 = 28 g

The FP for a serving of wheat-based pasta (spaghetti) is 28 grams indicating that 28 grams of carbohydrate are not leaving your intestine and can potentially cause bacterial overgrowth, gas and reflux. This is the real reason so many people get heartburn from eating spaghetti. The rice-based pasta on the other hand, gives a much more reasonable FP of 5 grams and is clearly the better choice. Note: The FP of rice pasta will depend on the type rice used in its production, which can be difficult to determine, as well as the production method and how long it was cooked. As I have indicated, some rices have more resistant starch than others. The rice pasta used was made from brown rice, which likely was relatively low in resistant starch.

Milk Comparison

Soy Milk (FP 2g) —*Less Potential for Heartburn*:
Serving size 8 oz, 224 g
NC 2 g
Fiber 1 g
GI 44
FP = ((100 – 44) x 2) / 100 + 1 = 2 g

Whole Milk (FP 8g) — *More Potential for Heartburn*:
Serving size 8 oz, 224 g
NC 11 g
Fiber 0 g
GI 27
FP = ((100 – 27) x 11) / 100 + 0 = 8 g

Comparing unsweetened soy milk to whole milk shows that soy milk will be much less apt to trigger heartburn symptoms. Skim milk fairs no better than whole milk and chocolate milk is worse with an FP of 11 g. These FP values make sense. The lactose in whole and skim milk and the additional sugar and fiber in the chocolate milk represent difficult-to-digest carbohydrates that are responsible for the higher FP values.

As you can see from these examples, fermentation potential depends less on the amount of carbohydrate in each food, and more on the difficulty of breaking down and absorbing different types of carbohydrates. Also note that glycemic index calculations are based on testing in healthy people who are not lactose-intolerant. This means that the FP value for milk would likely be higher if the glycemic index had been determined in lactose-intolerant people.

Now that we've taken a thorough look at fermentation potential, a key metric when trying to deal with the symptoms of GERD, it's time to look at how to incorporate this value into a diet plan that will change the way you eat and live. In the long run, a dietary approach to GERD, based on fine-tuning the inputs to the digestive process, is more likely to produce the results you're looking for.

Chapter 10: The Fast Tract Diet

On The Fast Tract

Now that you understand how difficult-to-digest carbohydrates can cause GERD symptoms, I'd like to introduce you to the most important element of my diet system for eliminating GERD symptoms — the Fast Tract Diet.

The goal of the Fast Tract Diet is to help you change your eating habits so that your digestive system breaks down and absorbs carbohydrates more efficiently. The better this process works, the less fermentable material is "left over" for bacterial fermentation, SIBO, and eventually GERD.

The diet's basic strategy is to limit foods with high FP values and replace them with foods with lower FP values. For example, we've looked at the benefit of replacing long grain rice varieties like Basmati with short grain Asian ("sticky") rice. Long grain rices (except jasmine rice) tend to have a very high amylose content (which is difficult to digest — and can cause heartburn) while short grain rices are higher in amylopectin (which is easy to digest — and won't cause heartburn).

There are three basic principles to keep in mind when evaluating FP values on your own.

Both low and high carbohydrate foods can have a low Fermentative Potential.

Fermentative Potential (FP) is the key measure regardless of the carbohydrate count.

Limiting foods with high FP will help control the overgrowth of bacteria in the small intestine — and acid reflux.

Though everyone is different, and able to tolerate varying amounts of difficult to digest carbohydrates, I recommend starting on the low end, consuming foods that are relatively low in FP.

Recommended FP total for a single meal:

FP between 0 and 10 is considered low.

FP between 10 and 15 is considered moderate.

FP equal or greater than 15 is considered high.

Recommended FP for a single day:

FP between 20 and 30 is considered low.

FP between 30 and 45 is considered moderate.

FP equal to or greater than 45 is considered high.

Make the Most of Your Diet

Before you get started with the recipes from the Meal Plans, let's look at some basic dietary practices that will help you make the Fast Tract Diet as effective as possible.

Minimize the Effects of Starches

There are several steps you can take to avoid consuming resistant starches. You can avoid starchy vegetables and fruits all together, but if you do include them in your diet, consume only fully ripened fruits and vegetables and fruits as they have lower amounts of resistant starch.

Make sure you eat only freshly prepared starchy vegetables (such as rice and potatoes). Cooked, then cooled, starchy vegetables can contain three times as much resistant starch. If you do consume leftover starches, heating them thoroughly helps gelatinize the retrograded starch.

Cook starchy vegetables well, because steaming, boiling or cooking starchy foods longer reduces the amount of resistant starch. This is important for potatoes, pasta, rice, and grains. You don't need to do this with non-starchy vegetables.

Avoid consuming whole grain products, as they are high in RS, and consider limiting or eliminating wheat products entirely until you determine their effect on you in a controlled manner (starting *after* your symptoms improve).

One piece of good news: Foods that don't contain carbohydrates, such as meats, fish, cheese, etc., have an FP value of zero and are not limited by the diet. Also, non-starchy vegetables (refer to Table 9 in Appendix B for a list of over 50 vegetables) have very low FP values — you can eat more of these foods more often!

Stay Hydrated

Drink plenty of water: at least six to eight glasses per day, especially if you are physically active. Water is required for the breakdown and metabolism of every food group as well as transporting nutrients and eliminating waste from your system. In addition, water is critical for maintaining body temperature, osmotic balance (controlling salt and

94

other electrolyte concentrations), blood pressure and normal bowel and bladder function.

Sometimes it's hard to remember to stay hydrated. I used to fill a glass with water, take a sip, and then forget about it. It's difficult to drink eight glasses a day one sip at a time! Later, I'd realize I was getting dehydrated. To improve my own water intake, I have started the habit of drinking at least one half of a glass of water as soon as I pour it.

I drink tap water, because the water in the Boston suburb where I live is of excellent quality and (lack of) taste. If it weren't, I would switch immediately to filtered or bottled water.

Other Liquids

While water is the most important component for staying hydrated, you can also enjoy a number of other liquids while on the Fast Tract Diet. During week one of the diet certain drinks are limited by amount. After the first week, however, drinks are only limited by the contributions of their FP values to your overall allowances.

You may be surprised to see coffee, tea and alcoholic drinks are allowed on the diet. I have found no convincing evidence that either caffeine or alcohol contributes to GERD symptoms. I believe that GERD symptoms associated with these drinks are actually caused by additives — for example, sucrose (table sugar) in coffee and tea, or sodas and drink mixes that contain high fructose corn syrup. Nevertheless, until you have your symptoms completely under control, I recommend that you limit caffeine-containing beverages to two per day and alcohol-containing beverages to one per day in the first week of the diet.

Also avoid sweetened wines, non-light beer, sweetened soft drinks, lactose-containing milk and milk products like non lactose-free ice cream, as well as all fruit juices. Here are some general guidelines:

> ### Water:
> *Unlimited: Six to eight glasses per day recommended to aid digestion.*
>
> ### Zero-calorie drinks including diet sodas:
> Not Allowed: *Soft drinks containing sugar.*
>
> Allowed: *Unlimited. But limit diet soft drinks to one can per day during week one and two.*

Caffeinated drinks such as tea and coffee:

Not Allowed: *Regular, fat free or low fat milk, sugar, half and half.*

Allowed: *Two cups per day with light cream, non-dairy creamer, lactose-free milk and Splenda, aspartame, or saccharin for a sweetener.*

Alcoholic drinks:

Not allowed: *Sweet wine, sugar sweetened drinks, and non-light beer.*

Allowed: *Light beer, dry (non-sweet) red or white wine, or mixed drinks made with non-sugar sweeteners and mixes; for example rum and diet coke. Limit to one drink per day during week one and limit to two drinks per day going forward until all symptoms are gone.*

Fruit Juices:

Not allowed: *During week one and week two.*

Allowed: *After week one and week two, they can be consumed within overall FP limits.*

Milk:

Not Allowed: *Lactose-containing milk.*

Allowed: *Light cream and lactose-free milk as used in recipes or within daily FP limits.*

Soy milk:

Not Allowed: *During week one.*

Allowed: *After week one, it can be consumed within overall FP limits.*

Vitamin and Mineral Supplements

Take a multivitamin daily that includes mineral. Vitamins B12, A, D, E, K and the minerals magnesium, calcium, iron, and zinc are important for digestive health. And your body's ability to use them can be affected by digestive malabsorption.

I take a generic multivitamin and mineral product that compares with Centrum every day. This supplement contains all the vitamins and minerals I just mentioned as well as lutein (a carotenoid antioxidant pigment from green leafy plants, egg yolks and animal fats) and lycopene (another carotenoid antioxidant pigment found in tomatoes and other fruits and vegetables). Your individual condition may require additional supplements. For example, you may want to take calcium if you're at risk for osteoporosis, or iron if you're affected by anemia (see note of caution below for iron).

Taking a combination multivitamin/mineral supplement along with specific calcium and fish oil supplements every day is a good way to make sure your body gets the nutrients you need — and that are often lacking in contemporary diets or depleted due to malabsorption.

Be cautious in using supplements, though. Iron, for example, can be toxic at high levels, and iron supplements should be used under a doctor's supervision. Some mineral supplements are not 100% pure. Calcium supplements, for instance, may contain other minerals including trace amounts of lead. Be sure to buy your supplements from reputable sources where the product is regularly tested by an accredited laboratory.

Healthy Lifestyle Choices

Avoid food and water poisoning. Both can wreak havoc on your digestive tract by upsetting the natural balance of your gut bacteria. I trust and prefer my home water supply, but when I travel, I tend to drink bottled water simply because I don't know where the local supply comes from or how it was processed, transported or stored. The same holds true for foods, or even for foods rinsed with water that you can't trust.

Exercise. Exercise accomplishes two goals. Body movements help keep your intestinal contents moving, but exercise also drives your body's demand for carbohydrates. This demand induces more enzyme production, more complete digestion, and more movement of sugars from your digestive tract into your blood stream. Exercise isn't a complete solution, though. Extreme sports, weight lifting and endurance running can result in reflux from exertion, shaking and other movements that put pressure on your stomach and lower esophageal sphincter.

On a positive note: Because the Fast Tract Diet allows some high-carb (and low-FP) foods, athletes who follow it can avoid the digestive symptoms sometimes associated with "carb loading" to increase glycogen storage.

Rest. Just one of the many reasons you need rest is that it helps your body have more energy for the hard work of digestion that requires strenuous, sustained and coordinated muscle contractions. Rest also reduces your stress level, the amount of acid your stomach produces between meals, and influences, if only indirectly, almost every aspect of your digestive process.

Fast periodically. Every few weeks or so, consume only water for several hours past your usual meal time, or even skip a meal entirely. Fasting gives your digestive system a break from the constant processing of food, giving it a chance to recover and prepare for more efficient digestion.

Slow down! How you eat is just as important as what you eat. Many of us race through our meals in an effort to save time for more pressing activities. But fast and furious eating is a severe disadvantage for your body's ability to digest food.

Take smaller bites, eat slowly and chew well. Consider counting to 20 on each mouthful. The amylase enzyme in your saliva can only act on small particles of food and only works until the starch reaches your stomach — at which point the amylase is destroyed. If your salivary amylase doesn't have the time to do its job, you'll have to rely on the pancreatic amylase in your small intestine, which is capable of finishing off the digestive process, but not the entire job of breaking down starches. I would never eat bread, rice, potatoes, corn, other wheat or grain products or pasta without chewing each bit to completion. If I didn't, these foods would absolutely give me severe heartburn.

Address Contributing Conditions

If you continue to experience symptoms you may wish to review Chapters 6-8, where I discuss some of the underlying conditions that, aside from diet, could contribute to the development of SIBO and GERD. If you have been following the diet (faithfully) for a two or three weeks and your symptoms have not significantly improved, here are a few more possibilities:

You may have a specific condition promoting SIBO, and you may want to consult with your health care provider to try to identify the problem. Any of the conditions discussed, such as motility issues, recent antibiotic use, gastric acid reduction, immune impairment, recent food poisoning or intestinal infection etc., can lead to SIBO. So can specific digestive disorders such as celiac disease and Crohn's disease, as well as systemic disorders that affect digestion, including diabetes, cystic fibrosis, etc.

Diagnosing and treating such disorders may be an important part of the solution.

Food tolerance issues or enzyme deficiencies can also limit the effectiveness of the diet.

A gluten-free diet may be necessary to help control the symptoms and progression of celiac disease. Or a high-quality lactase enzyme supplement may be necessary to reduce SIBO-related symptoms for people who are lactose-intolerant but continue to eat foods that contain lactose.

People who have an amylase deficiency have trouble digesting even small amounts of starch, including resistant starch (mainly amylose) and even the normally easy-to-digest starch amylopectin. An amylase enzyme supplement can greatly increase the efficiency of starch digestion for these individuals including people with cystic fibrosis or pancreas problems that affect the digestion of starches. Also, to limit resistant starch, don't eat leftover refrigerated or frozen rice mentioned in the recipes as resistant starch can build up in cold storage. Though a little more difficult to make small portions of rice, try using only freshly made rice for each dish.

If you consume legumes, even in smaller amounts, you might consider taking Beano, a product that contains the enzyme alpha-d-galactosidase, before meals. This enzyme breaks down the complex sugars raffinose, stachyose and verbascose present in legumes down into simple sugars and sucrose that can be more efficiently digested and absorbed.

Probiotics

Probiotics are another alternative that can make it easier to digest carbohydrates. These products contain live microorganisms (usually freeze-dried) that are believed to improve intestinal or general health. Two common bacteria used in probiotics are *Lactobacillus acidophilus* and *Bifidobacterium bifidum*. *Bifidobacteria*, in particular, are very efficient at breaking down oligosaccharides such as lactose, sucrose, raffinose, and stachyose. The lactobacilli can help with break down lactose in the small intestine.[86]

Enthusiasts claim that probiotics can reduce cholesterol, lower blood pressure, improve IBS symptoms, strengthen the immune system, and help prevent cancer.

Personally, I have found the evidence for some of these health claims are mixed or non-existent. There are, however, reasons to think that they might help with SIBO-related conditions. The bacteria in probiotics do produce lactic acid and little or no carbon dioxide, which is healthy for your digestive tract. In most cases, the bacteria used as dairy starter cultures are homolactic fermenters (only make lactic acid as an end product), so you don't have to worry that they'll produce symptom-causing gas.

Only use high-quality probiotic supplements from reputable suppliers. Store them as directed. Take probiotics on a regular schedule as indicated on the label.

Monitor Your Progress

You may be wondering how long it takes to see results from this diet. For most people, GERD symptoms caused by over-consumption of difficult-to-digest carbohydrates should significantly improve over a period of one to three days (similar to the results reported in the clinical study of this diet in Chapter 1). Some conditions that involve more extensive damage to the cells that line the intestine (celiac or Crohn's disease, cystic fibrosis, etc.) may require more time for the mucosal surface to heal.

Tracking your diet and symptoms is one of the most powerful tools you have in treating SIBO-related conditions with the Fast Tract Diet. Make a list of any digestive symptoms you have before you start the diet. Check your progress every week to see whether the symptoms have begun to subside. Also, record your meals and snacks. In most cases, your symptoms should show improvement relatively quickly as you follow the diet, and you should be able to start checking symptoms off your list.

I've included a dietary journal template (Appendix C) to help you track the foods you eat and your symptoms. The journal can help you identify specific foods (lactose, fructose, starches, fiber, etc.) that affect you.

Once your symptoms have greatly improved or disappeared, you can consider adding back some favorite foods you've had to avoid. Make these changes gradually, and keep careful track of how your digestive tract responds. Try not to increase different kinds of difficult to digest carbohydrates — for example, fructose and lactose — at the same time. Again, this gradual approach requires knowing which foods contain which carbohydrates. Separate any changes you make by at least a few days so that you can identify which changes affect your symptoms.

Next Steps

For most people, the solution may be as simple as refocusing your efforts on following the diet — and eating fewer foods, particularly the five difficult-to-digest carbohydrates discussed in this book. Changing your diet can be difficult. Business travel, restaurant dining, dinner with friends, or even your own preferences may make it difficult to stick to your resolutions. If you fall into this category, simple behavior-change strategies like keeping a food journal, giving yourself tangible incentives, or just clearing the foods you should avoid out of your refrigerator and pantry are more likely to succeed than simple will power.

Chapter 11: The Fast Tract Plan

For your first two weeks on the diet, I recommend following the Week One and Week Two Meal Plans contained in Appendix A. They contain recipes for every meal, snack and dessert you'll need for those first weeks. They'll help you improve your symptoms immediately, while you gain experience preparing low-FP recipes.

The recipes in the meal plans represent a blend of traditional American and Japanese foods. The ingredients include fresh seafood, beef, chicken and pork, a wide variety of vegetables, soy-based foods like tofu, and low-amylose starches like Russet Burbank potatoes and jasmine or sticky rice. All of the ingredients are easy to digest and absorb because they possess low fermentative potential values. And they are easy to find in your local market or, for a few items, a grocery store that carries Asian foods.

Preparing Recipes and Weighing Foods

The recipes are easy to prepare, and pretty much self-explanatory. Just make sure you use the specific kinds of food listed in the recipes without substitutions, particularly with regard to starches.

Ingredient amounts and serving sizes are listed in ounces and grams. I recommend buying a good kitchen, dict, or shipping scale that is accurate from a pound or two down to less than an ounce. Not only do you want to make sure that you're preparing the recipes properly, but serving sizes will often need to be adjusted (downward) to make FP limits. The scale will help you check and/or modify recipes, especially as you begin to develop your own.

Meal Plans for Week One and Week Two

I have developed complete meal plans — including meals, snacks, and desserts — for the first two weeks of the diet (see Appendix A) to make it as easy as possible for you to get started.

Both the Week One and Week Two Meal Plans include seven breakfast, seven lunch, and seven dinner choices, as well as snacks and desserts. Some of the recipes make one or two servings, while others are written for more (such as quiche, turkey dinner, or lasagna). In each case, the ingredient amounts can be adjusted accordingly to the number of desired servings — or leftovers can be refrigerated or frozen.

Both plans are based on the low-FP approach proven to be effective in the clinical study discussed in chapter 1. The average daily FP level is approximately 30 grams.

You can also use the meal plans and recipes to develop a shopping list to make sure you have all of the foods and ingredients you need on hand. During these first two weeks, make every effort to eat only the meals, snacks and desserts listed in the meal plan. The more you stick to the plan, the better your chances of getting results.

The Meal Plans provide specific instructions on allowed drinks. Note the limit of two caffeinated drinks and one alcoholic drink per day during this first week. Also note that certain drinks, sweeteners, mixes and certain types of wine are not allowed. After week one, alcoholic drinks are only limited by the FP guidelines for beer, wine and mixes as alcohol itself does not contribute to FP (though it may have a slight effect on glycemic index and therefore FP).

The Week One Meal Plan does not include foods that contain wheat. Wheat products often contain significant amounts of resistant starch and can be a factor in some people's GERD symptoms. Some condiments, such as soy sauce, used in the meal plan recipes may contain small amounts of gluten, but in each case, gluten-free products are available if you suspect you are intolerant of even small amounts of gluten. For most people, this will not be necessary.

The Week Two Meal Plan contains a few wheat products, providing an opportunity to check whether this leads to an increase in your symptoms. After week two, you may consume wheat-containing products — in accordance with FP limits — to determine if your own digestive system can tolerate these foods.

Follow up

After the first week on the diet, I would expect you to have experienced significant improvement in your symptoms. If so, you should move on to the Week Two Meal Plan. If not, you should ask yourself the following questions:

> *Did I follow the meal plan and recipes exactly?*

> *Did I consume any additional carbohydrates (including wheat products, desserts, medicines, supplements, candy, cough syrup, drinks etc.) that might have caused my symptoms to persist?*

> *Was I practicing the healthy digestion techniques outlined in previous chapters such as eating slowly, chewing each bite*

extremely well, taking any needed supplements such as lactase if lactose intolerant, drinking enough water, exercising to improve peristalsis, etc.?

Do I suffer from an underlying condition that increases my reflux symptoms that requires diagnosis and treatment? (Refer to chapter 6.)

Are the types of food I prepared truly equivalent to the low FP foods recommended in the Week One Meal Plan?

For instance, did I use short grain glutinous rice (or jasmine rice) instead of the high-FP varieties? It's important to follow the recipe for preparing this kind of rice closely to make sure the result is soft and fluffy, with a low FP. As an alternative, you can buy freshly-prepared sticky rice from a reputable sushi restaurant.

Once you've identified and eliminated these obstacles to the effectiveness of the diet, you're ready to try the Week One Meal Plan again. This time, consider lowering your daily FP level to 25 grams per day. For instance, you may want to consume fewer mixed nuts, which, though low in net carbs, contain significant amounts of fiber, which adds to FP. Another approach is to replace the rice in the meal plans with low FP vegetables, as the type of rice or the way it's being prepared or stored can generate resistant starch. You might also want to cut carbohydrates across the board to see if you can identify the "fuel" driving your symptoms. Remember, the key is in the carbs, not the proteins or fats.

Once you've gotten results — in the form of reduced symptoms — from the Week One Plan, it's time to move on to the Week Two Plan. By the end of the second week, you'll have learned how to prepare a wide variety of low-FP foods.

You'll find that you're consulting the FP tables in Appendix B regularly.

First, you can use them to determine foods and serving sizes that fit your target FP values for each meal and for each day.

One good first step is to set a daily limit on total FP for each day. I recommend keeping your total FP grams per day under forty for the first few weeks.

When you're developing your own daily plans, choose serving sizes that seem reasonable, and then check the FP value. If necessary, adjust the serving sizes to meet your FP goal.

For example, let's say that you have already consumed an FP of 33 grams for the day, but want to have a piece of chocolate for dessert. The tables list 1.6 ounces (44 grams) of chocolate as having an FP value of 15 grams. If you want to keep your daily FP under 40 grams, you'll need to reduce the serving size of the chocolate. In this case, you could only eat about one half the amount or 0.8 ounces (22 grams) to limit FP to 7.5 grams. If your piece of chocolate weighed 1.6 ounces (about the size of a Hershey bar), you could just break it in half — or you could actually weigh it on a scale.

Or, if you want to have blueberries and cream but you only have 6 FP grams available for dessert, just reduce the amount from the 120 gram serving size listed in the table (FP 10 grams) to 74 grams (1/2 cup) which has an FP of 5 grams. One-quarter cup of cream would add 1 FP gram for a total of 6 grams.

The tables can also serve as a good source for creating shopping lists. For instance, before shopping for fruits, notice that the low-FP fruits include: watermelon, cantaloupe, dates, strawberries, pineapple, peaches, lychee and apricots. Other berries and fruits are acceptable, but only in limited amounts.

It might help to do a quick scan of the tables and familiarize yourself with the foods at the top of each table (low-FP, heartburn-friendly) and the foods at the bottom of each table (high-FP, less heartburn-friendly). Notice that some tables, such as table 9 (for vegetables) contain mostly low-FP, heartburn-friendly foods, while other tables, such as table 7 (for pasta) contain mostly high-FP heartburn-unfriendly foods.

Creating Your Own Recipes

At some point you'll probably feel the urge to create your own new recipes. One relatively easy way is to adapt the existing recipes with new ingredients or in new combinations.

Whether adapting existing recipes or creating entirely new recipes, you'll follow the same Fermentative Potential (FP) guidelines used to develop the Week One and Week Two Meal Plans. This way, your new recipes are unlikely to cause new or recurring symptoms.

Again, you'll need to consult the FP tables in Appendix B. These tables contain FP values for over 300 different types of food. The FP tables are based on food types and list serving sizes in both ounces and grams.

Use your scale to check and adjust your ingredients against the values in the tables. You can also compare to the values given for the existing recipes. (Note that the serving sizes in the tables were chosen for uniformity in comparing FP values.)

What About Foods That Aren't Listed?

There are several reasons that specific foods may not be listed in the FP tables. These include:

1. The glycemic index value, required to calculate the FP value, may not exist. This could be because the food has so few carbs that the test cannot be done. (Or people can't eat enough of the food to reach the 50 grams of carbs needed for the test.)

In most cases, this means that the food doesn't contain enough carbs to be a threat and you can eat them without much concern. In many of these cases, such as low-carb vegetables, I have approximated an FP value based on an estimated GI. (The average GI for known vegetables is 62. An estimated GI of 50 for vegetables is conservative and errs on the side of caution).

2. The food is not very common and no one has thought (or paid) to perform the GI test on the food.

3. The food has no carbs. In this case, that also means that the FP is zero and you can consume it without limit. I have included some of these foods such as meats, cheeses, and seafood.

4. The food is not common to North America and including it would be of limited value.

In the case of 2 and 4, the GI can be estimated based on similar foods and an estimated FP can then be calculated. The best approach in these cases is to err on the side of caution with a lower GI estimate giving a higher FP.

In cases where you cannot find the food in the FP tables, determine whether there are appreciable carbs in the food. If not, the food can be considered safe to consume in normal quantities. If you find a food that is not in the tables, but you are able to find the GI value, serving size, net carbs and fiber levels for the food, you can calculate the FP value yourself using the formula for FP given below:

$$FP = \frac{(100 - GI)xNC}{100} + DF + SA$$

As a reminder: To calculate FP, you plug in the values for net carbs (NC), dietary fiber (DF), sugar alcohols (SA), and the glycemic index (GI) for each food. Now you can calculate the fermentation potential. If there are no sugar alcohols or fiber, the values for those variables are zero.

Appendix A: Meal Plans and Recipes

109

Week One Fast Tract Diet Plan

DAY 1 — Daily FP 43 grams

Breakfast: **Morning Berry Smoothie — Serves 1 — FP 8 grams**

  ½ cup strawberries (or blueberries)

  ½ cup plain unsweetened yogurt

  ½ cup light cream

  1 tablespoon (or to taste) Splenda

Combine all ingredients in a blender. Blend until smooth. Serve chilled.

NOTE: Additionally, you can have up to 2 ounces cheese, 2 strips of breakfast meets (bacon, sausage, ham, etc.) or a hardboiled egg if desired.

Lunch: **Hot Chicken Wings — Serves 1 — FP 4 grams**

  ¾ pounds chicken wings.

  2 tablespoons blue cheese dressing

  2 large stocks of celery cut in 4 inch lengths

   1 melon wedge

Broil chicken wings at medium to high heat for about 30 minutes or until fully cooked. Coat chicken wings with buffalo wing sauce (Ken's Steakhouse wing sauce is a good choice). Serve with blue cheese dressing, celery and melon wedge. Alternatively, season with salt in pepper if you don't want hot wings.

Snack: **Sweetened Nut Mix — Makes 8 daily servings — FP 14 grams per daily 3 ounce serving**

  1 ½ pounds of mixed nuts (6 ounces each of pecans,

walnuts, cashews, and pecans)

1 egg white, beaten until frothy

1 ½ tablespoons of butter, melted in microwave and cooled

¾ cup Splenda

¾ teaspoon sea salt

2 teaspoons ground cinnamon

1 teaspoon vegetable oil

Beat egg white in large bowl. Blend in salt, Splenda, cooled butter, and cinnamon. Add nuts and mix to coat. Spread the mixture on a large oiled baking pan and bake at 260 degrees for 45 minutes stirring each 15 minutes. Allow mix to cool and store in an airtight container.

Note: 3 ounces of snack mix is allowed for each day. I recommend weighing out 3 ounce portions for each day and storing in separate baggies. The recipe makes eight days worth. (24 ounces divided by 8 days = 3 ounces per day.)

Dinner: Turkey, Squash and Green Beans — Serves 4 — FP 12 grams

One small turkey (under 10 pounds). Alternately, use

a small chicken for fewer servings

1 butternut squash, peeled

1 pound green beans, with ends trimmed

½ teaspoon Bell's Seasoning

1 tablespoons vegetable oil

Salt and pepper

Rub turkey (or chicken) with vegetable oil and pat with salt, pepper and Bell's seasoning. Cook turkey (or chicken) in oven preheated to 325 degrees for approximately 4 hours (one hour for chicken) or until meat thermometer indicates the meat is fully cooked. While turkey (or chicken) is cooling, prepare gravy from the drippings by simmering drippings with an equal part of water. Thicken with no more than one teaspoon of potato starch mixed to remove lumps with a small amount of cold water. Steam peeled squash and green beans separately until tender and add butter, salt and pepper. Slice the turkey and serve.

Note: Save the turkey carcass for the soup recipe.

Dessert: Cheesecake — Serves 8 — FP 5 grams

2 8 ounce containers of cream cheese, warmed to

room temperature

1 cup Splenda

3 large eggs

1 teaspoon vanilla extract

¾ cup heavy cream

Gently beat together all warmed ingredients, adding the eggs and cream gradually. Do not over-beat. Add the filling to pie crust (recipe below) and bake at 350 degrees for 1 hour. Cool and then refrigerate. Serve with Splenda-sweetened whipped cream (recipe below) and berries if desired. Freeze leftovers.

Almond Crust — Makes one pie

1 ½ cup ground almond flour

4 tablespoons Splenda

¼ cup butter, melted

Mix together almond flour, Splenda, and melted butter. Press the mixture into a greased 9-inch pie pan covering both the bottom and sides of the pan.

Whipped Cream — Serves 8

1 cup heavy cream, chilled

3 tablespoons Splenda

1 teaspoon vanilla extract

In a large mixing bowl, combine chilled cream, Splenda and vanilla extract. Set bowl inside a larger bowl filled with crushed ice. (To keep the cream chilled) Whip the cream with an electric mixer until light and fluffy.

DAY 2 — Daily FP 31 grams

Breakfast: Fried Eggs and Bacon — Serves 1 — FP 0 grams

2 eggs

4 slices bacon (or sausage)

Cook bacon (or sausage) in pan until crisp (browned). Remove from pan and drain on paper towel. Heat 1 teaspoon vegetable oil or butter in a pan at medium-high heat. Fry eggs over easy, sunny side up or scramble as preferred. Add a slice of cheese if desired. Serve eggs with the bacon.

Lunch: Chili Mayo Shrimp with Fresh Veggies — Serves 1 — FP 10 grams

3 romaine lettuce leaves, washed and dried

4 large shrimp (or 3 strips of cooked chicken breast)

2 cherry tomatoes

¼ English cucumber (or regular cucumber), sliced the long way into two-inch long "match sticks."

2 slices sweet onion

¼ cup celery, finely chopped

¼ avocado, peeled

¼ cup mayonnaise

2 tablespoons lemon juice

½ tablespoon chili sauce (use less for less spicy)

½ tablespoon ketchup

Salt

Bring four cups of water to a boil. Peel and de-vein the shrimp and boil for about 2 minutes. Rinse with cold water and chill. Mix mayonnaise, lemon juice, chili sauce and ketchup in a large bowl. Add salt to taste. Toss shrimp, celery, and cherry tomato halves with the dressing in the same bowl. Scoop the mixture onto large lettuce leaves. Garnish with English cucumber, avocado wedges and onion slices.

NOTE: Additionally, you can have 2 ounces of cheese.

Snack: Nut-Thins (Blue Diamond Brand) — Serves 1 — FP 12 grams

Limit serving to 8 crackers. Add cheese, meats, pickles if preferred.

Dinner: Grilled Steak, Mushrooms and Broccoli — Serves 1 — FP 6 grams

1 rib eye (or similar) grilling steak

5 large mushrooms, sliced in half

1 cup broccoli crowns, sliced

1 tablespoon olive oil

2 teaspoons butter

Salt and pepper

Pat steaks with salt and pepper. Grill or broil steaks until medium rare or desired doneness. Coat mushrooms with olive oil and add salt and pepper (this can be done in a plastic bag or bowl. Grill or sauté mushrooms until tender. Steam broccoli until tender. Add 2 tablespoons butter, salt and pepper. Serve.

Dessert: Watermelon — Serves 1 — FP 3 grams

> 1 cup watermelon — diced.

Serve watermelon chilled.

DAY 3 — Daily FP 33 grams

Breakfast: Cottage Cheese, Melon and Hard Boiled Eggs — Serves 1 — FP 2 grams

> ½ cup cottage cheese
>
> ½ cup cantaloupe melon — diced
>
> 2 eggs
>
> Salt
>
> 1 teaspoon butter

Bring approximately eight cups of water to a boil. Carefully place egg(s) in the boiling water with a large spoon. Boil egg for 12 minutes. Carefully replace hot water with warm water. Serve salted, buttered eggs with cottage cheese and melon.

Lunch: Antipasto Salad — Serves 1 — FP 5 grams

> 2-3 cups leafy green lettuce, mixed greens or spinach
>
> 2 cherry tomatoes
>
> 2 mushrooms

1 artichoke heart (limit artichoke because of fructans)

4-6 black olives

1 pepperoncini (sweet pepper)

3-5 slices salami or ham, cut in quarters

1-2 ounces mozzarella cheese, cut in strips

2 tablespoons olive oil

1 tablespoon white or regular balsamic vinegar

Toss the greens with a mixture of olive oil and balsamic vinegar in a large serving bowl. Top with vegetables, meats and mozzarella cheese strips. Serve.

NOTE: Alternatively, use bottled Italian or Greek dressing.

Snack: Spiced Nut Mix — 3 Ounces Serves 1 — FP 14 grams

3 cups Rice Chex cereal

9 cup mixed nuts

3 tablespoons butter

2 tablespoons Worcestershire sauce

1-½ teaspoons seasoned salt

¾ teaspoon garlic powder

½ teaspoon onion powder

Combine Rice Chex and nuts in a large microwavable bowl. Melt butter in microwave for about 25 seconds. Add spices and Worcestershire sauce to melted butter and oil, mix and add to snack mix. Mix combination with large spoon. Heat in microwave on high for six minutes, pausing to mix every two minutes. Spread on paper towels to cool, about 20 minutes. Serve or store in an airtight container.

Note: I recommend weighing out 3 ounce portions for each day and storing in separate baggies. You can use either the salty snack recipe or the Sweet Nut Mix recipe. In both cases, 3 ounces per day are allowed.

Dinner: Miso Cod with Rice and Squash — Serves 1 — FP 7 grams

1 Cod fish fillet, approximately ¾ pound (or other

white fish)

1 teaspoon miso paste (fermented soy product, Asian

grocery)

1 teaspoon rice wine

½ teaspoon Splenda

1 lemon wedge, squeezed

1 stem scallion, chopped

1 small zucchini squash, sliced the long way for

grilling

1 small summer squash, sliced the long way for

grilling

Rub fish with a small amount of vegetable oil. Sprinkle with one pinch of salt and pepper. Mix miso, rice wine, Splenda, lemon juice and scallions. Coat fish on top with miso dressing and broil for about 15-20 minutes on high in preheated oven. Remove from heat when the fish is fully cooked.

Coat squash with vegetable oil and salt and pepper. Grill squash (or roast in oven).

Serve fish with squash and ½ cup of rice (recipe below).

Asian Sticky Rice — Serves 5

1 cup rice

1 cup water

Prepare sticky rice in advance. Rinse rice with cold water three to four times or until water runs clear. Mix rice with water and soak for 10 minutes prior to cooking in a rice cooker. Turn on the rice cooker. Don't open the lid for approximately 25 minutes. Let the rice sit for another 10 minutes. Fluff rice prior to serving.

Note: Wrap left over rice tightly in plastic wrap and freeze. Heat left over rice in the microwave in the plastic wrap until steaming hot. Be careful removing plastic wrap to avoid burns.

Dessert: Ice Cream or Soy Creamy Frozen Dessert — FP 5 grams

½ cup lactose-free Breyers ice cream

Serve the ice cream adding a few nuts and berries if desired. Alternatively, serve ½ cup of Trader Joe's Soy Creamy Frozen Dessert. No other substitutions.

DAY 4 — Daily FP 23 grams

Breakfast: Morning Berry Smoothie — Serves 1 — FP 8 grams

½ cup strawberries (or blueberries)

½ cup plain unsweetened yogurt

½ cup light cream

1 tablespoon (or to taste) Splenda

Combine all ingredients in a blender. Blend until smooth. Serve chilled in a tall glass.

NOTE: Serve alone or with up to 2 ounces cheese, 2 strips of breakfast meets (bacon, sausage, ham, etc.) or a hardboiled egg if desired.

Lunch: Chicken Lettuce Wraps — Serves 2 — FP 3 grams

3 iceberg lettuce leaves

¼ English cucumber sliced the long way into two-inch long "match sticks."

1 pound chicken breast, chopped

1 scallion, chopped

1 tablespoons soy sauce

2 teaspoons Splenda

½ teaspoon rice vinegar

1/3 can water chestnuts, chopped

1 tablespoon vegetable oil

Mix soy sauce, rice vinegar and Splenda. Sauté chicken in vegetable oil until half cooked. Add water chestnuts and continue to sauté. Add soy sauce mixture just before chicken is fully cooked and continue to sauté. Mix in scallions and remove from heat. Place the chicken in the middle of a lettuce leaf, add a few cucumber sticks and roll. Dip the roll in the source to eat.

Peanut sauce

1 tablespoons creamy peanut butter

2 teaspoons rice wine

1 ½ teaspoons soy sauce

¼ teaspoon spicy sesame oil

2 teaspoons water

1 pinch dried red pepper

1.5 teaspoons Splenda

Combine all ingredients and mix.

Notes: Make sure the peanut butter is at room temperature before mixing. Halve the amount of spicy sesame oil and red pepper for a milder dish.

Snack: Celery with Cream Cheese — Serves 1 — FP 1 gram

Spread cream cheese onto two large celery stocks, cut in half and serve. Add sliced olives if desired.

Dinner: Pork Roast, Grilled Spinach and Cauliflower — Serves 3 — FP 6 grams

1 Pork tenderloin — about 1 ½ pounds

1 head cauliflower

1 bag (12 ounces) spinach

2 tablespoons vegetable oil

2 tablespoon butter

2 cloves garlic, thinly sliced

2 cloves of garlic, minced

1 tablespoon rosemary

1 tablespoon thyme

½ cup heavy cream

Salt and pepper

Preheat oven to 425 degrees. Rub pork tenderloin with one tablespoon of vegetable oil and pat with rosemary, thyme, minced garlic, salt and pepper. Bake at 425 degrees for approximately 30 minutes being sure the pork is fully cooked.

Steam cauliflower until extra soft. Remove from heat and whip with butter and cream using an electric mixer. Add salt and pepper to taste.

Sauté spinach and sliced garlic with one tablespoon olive oil. Add salt and pepper.

Remove pork roast from heat and let sit for 10 minutes before serving.

Dessert: Milk Chocolate — Serves 1 — FP 5 grams

½ ounce milk chocolate.

Do not substitute with dark chocolate. Dark chocolate has too much fiber. Limit serving to ½ ounce per person.

DAY 5 — Daily FP 39 grams

Breakfast: Spinach & Cheddar Cheese Omelet — Serves 1 — FP 2 grams

  2 eggs

  1 cup fresh raw spinach

  2 ounces cheddar cheese, grated

  4 teaspoons vegetable oil or butter

Sauté spinach with two teaspoons oil or butter in a pan until tender. Remove from pan. Heat remaining vegetable oil or butter in a pan at medium-high heat. Whisk eggs in a small bowl and pour them into the pan. Lift eggs at their edges with a spatula and tip the pan to make sure the egg mixture is cooked. Place spinach over the eggs and sprinkle with cheese. Turn the heat down to medium. Use your spatula to fold the omelet in half. Cook for 2-3 more minutes. Slide the omelet onto a plate. Serve it with the cooked meat.

NOTE: Serve alone or with up to 2 slices bacon or sausage.

Lunch: Turkey Soup with Rice — Serves 5 — FP 6 grams

  1 cooked turkey carcass (from turkey recipe)

2 sticks celery

1 sweet onion, chopped

1 medium carrot, sliced

6 medium mushrooms, sliced

½ teaspoon Bell's seasoning

Salt and pepper

Place turkey carcass with approximately ¾ of the meat removed (see cooked turkey recipe) into a large pot with approximately 3 quarts of water. Bring to a boil and simmer for several hours until the meat falls easily from the bone. Remove bones. Add salt, pepper and Bell's seasoning. Sauté onions, celery, carrots and mushrooms and add to soup. Continue to simmer the soup for another 30 minutes. Serve with ½ cup rice and salad.

Asian Sticky Rice — Serves 5

1 cup rice

1 cup water

While soup is simmering, prepare sticky rice. Rinse rice with cold water three to four times or until water runs clear. Mix rice with water and soak for 10 minutes prior to cooking in a rice cooker. Turn on the rice cooker. Don't open the lid for approximately 25 minutes. Let the rice sit for another 10 minutes. Fluff rice prior to serving.

Note: Wrap left over rice tightly in plastic wrap and freeze. Heat left over rice in the microwave in the plastic wrap until steaming hot. Be careful removing plastic wrap to avoid burns.

Tossed Salad — Serves 1

2 cups mixed greens

¼ tomato, cut into wedges

2 thin slices of onion

½ tablespoon balsamic vinegar

1 tablespoon olive oil

Salt and pepper

Rinse greens and spin dry in a salad spinner. Tear greens and toss them with olive oil and vinegar, pepper and salt. Add tomato wedges and sliced onions. Serve soup and rice with salad.

Snack: **Sweetened Nuts Mix —3 ounces Serves 1 — FP 14 grams**

Dinner: **Grilled Chicken, Broccoli Rabe and Squash — Serves 2 — FP 6 grams**

1 pound chicken thighs

2 tablespoons soy sauce

1 ½ teaspoons ginger, minced

1 ½ teaspoons garlic, minced

1 small bunch broccoli rabe (or 1 ½ cups broccoli)

1 acorn squash, peeled and diced with seeds

 removed

2 teaspoons vegetable oil

2 teaspoons butter

Salt and pepper

Marinate chicken thighs refrigerated for one hour in mixture of soy sauce, ginger, garlic and pepper. Grill chicken on medium-low grill until fully cooked (alternatively sauté). Trim broccoli rabe stems by 1 ½ inch. Sauté broccoli rabe (1/2 bunch at a time) in vegetable oil with pinch of salt and pepper until cooked. Steam squash until fully cooked. Add butter, salt and pepper and mash. Serve.

Dessert: Mixed Berries with Cream — Serves 1 — FP 11 grams

½ cup blueberries

½ cup strawberries, sliced

½ cup of light cream

2 teaspoons Splenda.

Mix berries with cream and add Splenda. Serve.

DAY 6 — Daily FP 33 grams

Breakfast: Ham Roll Ups with Cheese and Fruit Cup — Serves 1 — FP 6 grams

3 slices of ham (prosciutto or salami can substitute)

3 slices of American or cheddar cheese

Combine cheese and ham, roll up and cut into bite-sized pieces.

Fruit Cup — Serves 1

1/3 cup watermelon, diced

1/3 cup cantaloupe, diced

2 strawberries, sliced

1/3 cup blueberries

Combine fruit and serve with Ham Roll Ups.

Lunch: MeatBalls with Mixed Peppers — Serves 2 — FP 11 grams

  1 pound ground beef

  1 cup tomato sauce (Use a brand with the fewest

  overall carb count.)

  ½ pound mixed (green, yellow and red) peppers

  ¼ sweet onion, finely chopped

  2 medium mushrooms, finely chopped

  1 egg, beaten

  ¼ cup freshly grated parmesan cheese

  1 clove of garlic, crushed and chopped

  1 teaspoon dried basil (or 1 tablespoon fresh basil)

  ¼ teaspoons salt

  ¼ teaspoon pepper

  1 ½ teaspoon vegetable oil

  ½ teaspoon butter

Sauté sweet onion and mushrooms in oil and butter. Add garlic, basil, salt and pepper and continue to sauté for another minute. In a large bowl, add this mixture to the ground beef mix briefly and add beaten eggs. Mix well and form into meatballs. Preheat the oven to 325 degrees and bake meatballs until browned and well cooked, approximately 35 minutes.

Place meatballs in 1 cup of tomato sauce and heat until sauce begins to boil. While the sauce simmers, coat peppers with olive oil, salt and pepper. Grill peppers and serve with meatballs and sauce.

Note: Do not consume more than ½ cup of tomato sauce per serving.

Snack: One bag of popcorn — Serves 2 — FP 5 grams

Follow the microwave directions to prepare. Add more melted butter and salt if needed. For a taste more like kettle corn, add a tablespoon of Splenda. Do not consume more than ½ bag per person.

Dinner: Broiled Salmon, Sticky Rice and Asparagus — Serves 2 — FP 5 grams

> 1 pound salmon filet
>
> ½ pound asparagus
>
> 1 tablespoon soy sauce
>
> ½ tablespoon balsamic vinegar
>
> 1 orange wedge, squeezed
>
> 1 teaspoon pepper

Mix soy sauce, balsamic vinegar, orange juice and pepper. Marinate salmon in mixture for two to three hours. Broil salmon for 20 to 25 minutes on high until fully cooked. Tent with foil if the top begins to over-brown.

Snap off bottom of asparagus spears and coat with olive oil, salt and pepper. Grill (or sauté) until cooked.

Serve salmon with asparagus and ½ cup of rice.

Asian Sticky Rice — Serves 5

> 1 cup rice
>
> 1 cup water

Prepare sticky rice in advance. Rinse rice with cold water three to four times or until water runs clear. Mix rice with water and soak for 10 minutes prior to cooking in a rice cooker. Turn on the rice cooker. Don't open the lid for approximately 25 minutes. Let the rice sit for another 10 minutes. Fluff rice prior to serving.

Note: Wrap left over rice tightly in plastic wrap and freeze. Heat left over rice in the microwave in the plastic wrap until steaming hot. Be careful removing plastic wrap to avoid burns.

Dessert: Ice Cream or Soy Ice Cream — FP 6 grams

½ cup lactose-free Breyers ice cream

or

½ cup Soy ice cream (Trader Joe's Soy Creamy Frozen

Dessert)

Serve the ice cream adding a few nuts and berries if desired.
No other ice cream substitutions allowed.

DAY 7 — Daily FP 36 Grams

Breakfast: Morning Berry Smoothie — Serves 1 — FP 8 grams

½ cup strawberries (or blueberries)

½ cup plain unsweetened yogurt

½ cup light cream

1 tablespoon (or to taste) Splenda

Combine all ingredients in a blender. Blend until smooth. Serve chilled.

NOTE: Additionally, you can have up to 2 ounces cheese, 2 strips of breakfast meets (bacon, sausage, ham, etc.) or a hardboiled egg if desired.

Lunch: Chef Salad — Serves 1 — FP 3 grams

2-3 cups iceberg or leafy green lettuce

2 cherry tomatoes

3 slices cucumber

2 slices green pepper

2 slices each of turkey and ham, sliced in strips

2 ounces mozzarella cheese

1 hard-boiled egg, quartered

4-6 black olives

2 tablespoons olive oil

1 tablespoon balsamic vinegar

Mix lettuce, tomatoes and combination of olive oil and balsamic vinegar in a large serving bowl. Layer meat, eggs and olives on top. Sprinkle on chopped nuts and cheese and serve.

NOTE: Alternatively, use Italian or Greek bottled dressing.

Snack: Nut-Thins (Blue Diamond Brand) with Hard Salami and Cheese — FP 12 grams

Slice salami and cheese and serve with crackers. Limit to 8 crackers.

Dinner: Asian Style Chicken and Vegetable Sauté with Rice — Serves 2 — FP 7 grams

1 pound chicken breast, cubed

2 cups broccoli

½ sweet onion

6 mushrooms

4 teaspoons soy sauce

1 tablespoon oyster sauce

2 tablespoons vegetable oil

Salt and pepper

Mix soy sauce and oyster sauce and set aside. Sauté chicken in 1 tablespoon vegetable oil. When cooked, add the soy/oyster sauce mixture and stir. Sauté vegetables in 1 tablespoon of vegetable oil adding a pinch of salt and pepper during the process. Mix vegetables and chicken together and serve with ½ cup of sticky rice.

Asian Sticky Rice — Serves 5

1 cup rice

1 cup water

Prepare sticky rice in advance. Rinse rice with cold water three to four times or until water runs clear. Mix rice with water and soak for 10 minutes prior to cooking in a rice cooker. Turn on the rice cooker. Don't open the lid for approximately 25 minutes. Let the rice sit for another 10 minutes. Fluff rice prior to serving.

Note: Wrap left over rice tightly in plastic wrap and freeze. Heat left over rice in the microwave in the plastic wrap until steaming hot. Be careful removing plastic wrap to avoid burns.

Dessert: Fruit Cup — Serves 1

1/3 cup watermelon, diced

1/3 cup cantaloupe, diced

2 strawberries, sliced

1/3 cup blueberries

Combine fruit and serve.

Week Two Fast Tract Diet Plan

DAY 8 — Daily FP 41 grams

Breakfast: **Spinach and Sausage Quiche — Serves 4 — FP 7 grams**

>6 large eggs
>
>½ pound Italian sausage
>
>1 cup fresh spinach, steamed, chopped and cooled
>
>½ bunch green onions, sautéed, chopped and cooled
>
>1 ½ cups cheddar or Monterey Jack cheese, shredded
>
>1 French baguette

Cook sausage completely at medium to medium-high heat and set aside. Whisk eggs until well blended. Add chopped green onions, spinach, shredded cheese and cooked sausage. Mix well. Pour mixture into pie crust (recipe below). Bake at 350 degrees for 45 minutes. Let cool for 10 minutes. While quiche is cooling, warm and slice the baguette. Serve the quiche with one piece of warmed baguette with butter.

Almond Crust — makes one quiche

>1 cup ground almond flour (thinner crust OK for quiche)
>
>3 tablespoons butter, melted

Mix together almond flour and melted butter. Press the mixture into a greased 8 or 9-inch pie pan covering both the bottom and sides of the pan.

Limit baguette to one piece, eat slowly and chew it well. Baguettes have a relatively low FP compared to other breads, but if this meal gives you heartburn, skip the baguette for now. As your system heals you may be able to add it back. Try again in one week.

Note: Can make this dish in advance and refrigerate or freeze for quick breakfasts.

Lunch: Antipasto Salad — Serves 1 — FP 7 grams

> 2 cups leafy green lettuce, mixed greens or spinach
>
> 2 cherry tomatoes
>
> 2 mushrooms
>
> 1 artichoke heart
>
> 3 black olives
>
> 3 green olives
>
> 1 pepperoncini (sweet pepper)
>
> ¼ avocado, peeled and cut into wedges
>
> 3 slices each of salami and prosciutto, rolled up
>
> 1-2 ounces mozzarella cheese, cut in strips or sliced
>
> 2 tablespoons olive oil
>
> 1 tablespoon white or regular balsamic vinegar

Toss the greens with a mixture of olive oil and balsamic vinegar in a large serving bowl. Top with vegetables and arrange meats and mozzarella cheese strips on the edge. Serve.

NOTE: Alternatively, use bottled Italian or Greek dressing.

Snack: Sweet Nut Mix (See recipe on Day 1) — FP 14 grams

Limit to 3 ounces per day.

Dinner: Barbecued Baby Back Ribs — Serves 4 — FP 8 grams

> 3 pounds pork baby back ribs (or pork spare ribs)
>
> 6 ounces fresh pineapple

Collard greens (recipe below)

Coleslaw (recipe below)

2 tablespoons vegetable oil

3 green onions

Rub — spice mix (recipe below)

Braising liquid (recipe below)

Rub Spice Mix

2 teaspoons dark brown sugar

1 tablespoon chili powder

1 teaspoon cumin

1 ½ tablespoon smoked paprika

1 ½ teaspoons salt

1 teaspoons black pepper

½ teaspoon cayenne pepper

Mix all ingredients except the ribs. Rub/pat the mixture onto the ribs and refrigerate for 2 hours to overnight.

Braising Liquid

1 cup white wine

2 tablespoons white wine vinegar

1 tablespoon Worcester sauce

1 teaspoon honey

2 garlic cloves, chopped.

Mix all the ingredients and refrigerate the braising liquid.

Preheat the oven to 350 degrees. Place the ribs in foil with the edges folded up to hold liquid. Add the braising liquid around the base of the ribs and cover tightly with another piece of foil. Braise the ribs at 350 degrees for one hour. Lower the temperature to 250 degrees and continue braising for 2 more hours. Remove the braising liquid and simmer over medium high heat to reduce the volume by about two thirds. Grill (Or broil) for about 10 minutes on each side on low heat basting with the braising liquid each time the ribs are turned.

Place medium sized pineapple chunks on skewers and grill for a few minutes on each side. Remove ribs and pineapple from grill. Sprinkle ribs with chopped green onions, salt and pepper.

Collard Greens — Serves 4

6 cups collard greens, chopped

2 ½ tablespoons vegetable oil

1 ½ cup chicken broth

½ teaspoon garlic powder

½ teaspoon onion powder

Salt and pepper

Sauté collard greens in vegetable oil on high heat with salt and pepper. Add chicken broth, garlic and onion powder and continue to cook on medium heat for 15 minutes.

Coleslaw — Serves 4

½ head green cabbage, washed and finely chopped

1 small carrot, shredded

¼ cup mayonnaise

¼ cup sour cream

2 tablespoons white vinegar

1 teaspoons lemon juice

1 teaspoon Dijon mustard

1 pinch salt and pepper

1 teaspoon Splenda

Mix cabbage with shredded carrots in a large bowl. Combine the remaining ingredients in a separate bowl and blend until smooth. Pour this dressing over the cabbage and carrots and toss until evenly coated.

Serve the ribs with pineapple, collard greens and coleslaw.

Dessert: Cheesecake — Serves 1 — FP 5 grams

Thaw one slice of cheesecake from Day One recipe. Add whipped cream — see day 1 recipe.

DAY 9 — Daily FP 27 grams

Breakfast: Tofu and Sausage — Serves 2 — FP 3 grams

8 ounces (1/2 block) tofu

8 ounces Italian sausage, sliced

2 green onions, finely chopped

2 teaspoons soy sauce

Pepper to taste

Hot chili sauce

4 large strawberries

1 teaspoon Splenda

Brown the sausage at medium-high heat until almost cooked. Cut tofu into ½ inch squares and add to sausage and sauté the mixture together until tofu becomes golden. Try to keep the tofu squares intact while cooking. Add the soy sauce (aim for the tofu as the sausage is already salty), chopped green onions and pepper and remove from heat. Serve with hot chili sauce and two strawberries sprinkled with Splenda on the side.

Lunch: Beef and Vegetable Soup with Rice — Serves 6 — FP 3 grams

2 pounds beef stew meat, such as shoulder roast

1 sweet onion, chopped

7 large mushrooms, quartered

2 stalks celery, chopped

1 large (or medium) carrot, thickly sliced

2 tablespoons vegetable oil

3 bay leaves

3 garlic cloves, crushed and chopped

Salt and pepper

Cut beef into cubes and brown at medium high heat with 1 tablespoon of vegetable oil. Set aside. Add 1 tablespoon of vegetable oil and sauté the chopped onions, celery, mushrooms, garlic and carrots on medium high heat for about 6 minutes. Place beef and vegetable mixture along with two to three bay leaves in a crock pot or large pan. Add just enough water to cover the mixture and let simmer for three hours (in pan) or six to eight hours (in a crock pot). Add salt and pepper to taste. Some people prefer a little curry to spice it up. Serve with ½ cup of rice (recipe below).

Asian Sticky Rice — Serves 5

1 cup rice

1 cup water

While the beef is simmering, prepare the sticky rice. Rinse rice with cold water three to four times or until water runs clear. Mix rice with water and soak for 10 minutes prior to cooking in a rice cooker. Turn on the rice cooker. Don't open the lid for approximately 25 minutes. Let the rice sit for another 10 minutes. Fluff rice prior to serving.

Snack: Yogurt with Berries — Serves 1 — FP 8 grams

½ cup yogurt

½ cup raspberries, blackberries or strawberries)

1 tablespoon Splenda

Mix yogurt with berries and sprinkle with Splenda to taste.

Dinner: Scallops, Asparagus and Jasmine Pilaf — Serves 2 — FP 8 grams

1 pound large scallops

3 parsley stems, finely chopped

1/3 lemon

1 teaspoon garlic, minced

10 asparagus spears

1 cup jasmine rice

1 ½ cups chicken broth

¼ red pepper, finely chopped

2 tablespoons butter

2 tablespoons olive oil

¼ cup white wine

Salt and pepper

Bring chicken both to a boil. Add rice and red pepper and stir. Simmer for 15 without lifting lid.

Place butter, 1 tablespoon olive oil and garlic in a pan on medium high heat. Add scallops with salt and pepper and sauté on both sides. Add white wine and continue to cook. When scallops are fully cooked, squeeze lemon juice over scallops and sprinkle parsley over the top.

Sauté asparagus with 1 tablespoon olive oil. Add salt and pepper to taste.

Serve scallops and asparagus with up to ¾ cup of jasmine rice. (A little more rice is OK at this point if your symptoms are under control. Otherwise stick with a ½ cup serving).

Dessert: **Key Lime Pie — Serves 8 — FP 5 grams**

4 egg yolks, beaten

1-¾ cups light cream

½ cup lime juice (about 4 limes, key limes are not

necessary)

3 teaspoons lime zest (gratings of skin of the lime)

4 tablespoons Splenda

2 cups whipped cream (Refer to Day 1 recipe)

Almond crust (recipe below)

Preheat the oven to 375 degrees. Combine the egg yolks, cream, lime juice, lime zest and Splenda and mix. Pour the mixture into the unbaked pie crust (recipe below) and bake for 12 to 15 minutes. Remove and cool, then refrigerate. Add whipped cream and serve with a lime wedge.

Almond Crust — makes one pie

1 ½ cup ground almond flour

4 tablespoons Splenda

¼ cup butter, melted

Mix together almond flour, Splenda, and melted butter. Press the mixture into a greased 9-inch pie pan covering both the bottom and sides of the pan.

It takes about 15 key limes to make ½ cup of key lime juice. Substituting 4 regular limes seems to work fine.

DAY 10 — Daily FP 27 grams

Breakfast:

Baked Ham and Asparagus Frittata — Serves 2 — FP 5 grams

4 eggs

½ cup ham, diced (or sausage)

¾ cup parmesan (or cheddar) cheese, grated

½ cup asparagus, chopped

1 tablespoon vegetable oil

1 slice white bread

1 teaspoon butter

Heat the oven to 400 degrees. Sauté ham and asparagus until cooked al dente. Whisk together eggs and ½ cup of cheese. Add the ham and asparagus and pour into several paper or foil-lined muffin tin cups about half way to the top (eggs will stick even to oil coated nonstick muffin tins). Sprinkle the remaining grated cheese over the top, add salt and pepper and bake for about 15 minutes until the top begins to brown. Serve with one piece of white toast and butter.

Lunch: **Shrimp Fried Rice — Serves 6 — FP 7 grams**

> 1 pound medium to large shrimp, fresh or frozen
>
> 4 cups prepared Asian sticky rice (recipe below)
>
> 2 eggs, beaten
>
> 2 scallions, chopped
>
> 3 tablespoons soy sauce
>
> 3 tablespoons vegetable oil
>
> 1 tablespoon butter
>
> Salt and pepper
>
> Avocado and Boston Lettuce Salad (recipe below)

Sauté whole shrimp in a hot pan with two tablespoons vegetable oil and two teaspoons of butter as well as salt and pepper until almost done. Add the rice (recipe below) to shrimp and continue to sauté. Move the mixture to one side and drop the eggs into the pan. Scramble the eggs quickly, and combining with the rice just before the eggs are fully cooked. Add chopped scallions to the mixture and drizzle 2 tablespoons soy sauce around the edge of the pan. Stir egg and soy sauce into the mixture. Serve with salad.

Asian Sticky Rice

> 1 ½ cup rice
>
> 1 ½ cup water

Prepare sticky rice in advance. Rinse rice with cold water three to four times or until water runs clear. Mix rice with water and soak for 10 minutes prior to cooking in a rice cooker. Turn on the rice cooker. Don't open the lid for approximately 25 minutes. Let the rice sit for another 10 minutes. Fluff rice prior to serving.

Note: Wrap left over rice tightly in plastic wrap and freeze. If you use leftover rice for this recipe, microwave to warm before adding to the pan.

Avocado and Boston Lettuce Salad — Serves 4

1 avocado, peeled and sliced

1 head Boston (Bibb) lettuce

2 strips cooked bacon, finely chopped

2 stems curly parsley, finely chopped

1/8 small sweet onion, finely chopped

4 tablespoons vegetable oil

3 tablespoons white balsamic vinegar

Salt and pepper

Add washed lettuce to individual salad bowls and cover with bacon and avocado slices. Mix oil with vinegar, salt, pepper, chopped onions and parsley. Pour dressing over salad.

Snack: **Pork Rinds and Onion Dip — Serves 2 — FP 0 grams**

Serve store bought pork rinds snack with onion dip prepared from mixing dehydrated onion soup mix with sour cream according to the directions on the onion soup mix package.

Dinner: **Eggplant Lasagna — Serves 8 - 10 — FP 9 grams**

1 medium eggplant (three cups)

1 ½ pounds mozzarella cheese, grated

2 cups whole milk ricotta cheese

28 ounces tomato sauce (bottled OK, look for sugar free, lowest carb brand)

1 cup green Bell pepper, chopped

½ cup onion, chopped

3 garlic cloves

1 pound sausage, browned and chopped

1 pound ground beef, browned

Salt and pepper

Salad (see recipe and ingredients below)

Brown the meat and sauté the vegetables and garlic. Mix the meat, tomato sauce and vegetables together. Slice the eggplant thin (this helps to keep the eggplant taste in check). Spread a thin coat of meat and sauce mix in a large baking dish. Add new layers of eggplant, sauce mix, mozzarella, and ricotta cheese. Repeat until all ingredients are used. Top with a layer of cheeses and salt and pepper. Bake at 350 degrees for about 45 minutes to an hour. Let cool for ten to fifteen minutes.

Tossed Salad — Serves 1

2 cups mixed greens

¼ tomato, cut into wedges

2 thin slices of onion

½ tablespoon balsamic vinegar

1 tablespoon olive oil

Salt and pepper

Rinse greens and spin dry in a salad spinner. Tear greens and toss them with olive oil and vinegar, pepper and salt. Add tomato wedges and sliced onions.

Serve lasagna with salad. I usually double the quantities when I make lasagna. You can chill and cut the leftovers into single serving pieces for heartburn-free lunches or warm and easy-to-serve dinners. Or freeze it for future meals.

Dessert: Pineapple Macaroons — Serves 5 — FP 6 grams

> 2 cups unsweetened shredded coconut
>
> 2 ounce fresh pineapple, finely chopped
>
> ½ cup egg whites
>
> 1 stick of butter, melted
>
> 1 teaspoon vanilla or almond extract
>
> 1 cup Splenda

Preheat oven to 325 degrees. Whip egg whites, vanilla extract and melted then cooled butter together. Mix in coconut, pineapple and Splenda. Spoon onto baking sheet covered with foil coated with oil. Bake for approximately 15 minutes, checking regularly. The recipe makes about 15 cookies. Three cookies per serving.

DAY 11 — Daily FP 33 grams

Breakfast: Morning Berry Smoothie — Serves 1— FP 8 grams

> ½ cup strawberries (or blueberries)
>
> ½ cup plain unsweetened yogurt
>
> ½ cup light cream
>
> 1 tablespoon (or to taste) Splenda

Combine all ingredients in a blender. Blend until smooth. Serve chilled.

NOTE: Additionally, you can have up to 2 ounces cheese, 2 strips of breakfast meets (bacon, sausage, ham, etc.) or a hardboiled egg if desired.

Lunch: Tri-Salad — Serves 2 — FP 7 grams

6 ounces tuna, packed in water

6 ounces chicken, cooked and chopped

2 hard-boiled eggs, chopped

3 tablespoons mayonnaise

3 tablespoons celery, finely chopped

6 large lettuce leaves

½ avocado, peeled and cut in wedges

½ tomato, sliced

Salt and pepper

Prepare two hard-boiled eggs by cooking them in boiling water for 12 minutes. Remove from heat, rinse in cold water and chill before using. Make separate tuna, chicken and egg salad mixtures by adding 1 tablespoon mayonnaise and 1 tablespoon celery to each. Add salt and pepper to taste. Serve 1 scoop of each mixture over 2 lettuce leaves. Serve with avocado and tomato wedges.

You can use either leftover or canned chicken in this dish. You may want to prepare a half-dozen hardboiled eggs and save four. Hard-boiled eggs make tasty heartburn-friendly snacks. Serve peeled and halved with salt and pepper.

Snack: Sweet Nut Mix (See recipe from Day 1) — FP 14 grams

Limit to 3 ounces per day.

Dinner: Chicken Piccata — Serves 4 — FP 3 grams

2 pounds boneless chicken thighs

½ cup zucchini squash, diced

½ cup yellow squash, diced

½ cup red pepper, diced

½ cup onion, diced

2 eggs

¼ cup soy sauce

¼ cup mayonnaise

3 tablespoons olive oil

1 tablespoon butter

¼ cup parsley (or 2 teaspoons dried parsley)

Salt and pepper

Cut chicken into pieces about 1 inch square. Sprinkle with salt and pepper. Beat two eggs. Coat the chicken with the egg mixture and pan fry with 1 tablespoon butter and 1 tablespoon olive oil. Sprinkle the chicken with parsley. Prepare a mixture of equal parts soy sauce and mayonnaise for dipping the chicken pieces into.

Sauté vegetables together in medium hot pan in two tablespoons vegetable oil until they begin to brown.
Serve.

Note: Chicken Piccata makes a wonderful on-the-run snack food.

Dessert: **Rum Custard — Serves 6 — FP 1 gram**

5 eggs

2 ¼ cups heavy cream

2 tablespoons light rum (optional)

1 cup granular Splenda

2 teaspoons vanilla extract

½ teaspoon salt

1 teaspoon nutmeg

1 teaspoon cinnamon

Preheat the oven to 350 degrees. Pour boiling water into a large baking tray to come up about 1/3 to the top. Whisk eggs together with other ingredients except nutmeg and cinnamon. Pour mixture into an 8 x 8 inch baking dish and sprinkle nutmeg and cinnamon over the top. Set the baking dish inside a baking tray making sure the hot water comes up to the level of the custard in the baking dish. Bake for 45 minutes or until a knife inserted in the center comes out clean. Cool and chill to allow custard to set before serving.

DAY 12 — Daily FP 31 grams

Breakfast: **Mushroom, Ham and Feta Cheese Omelet — Serves 1 — FP 6 grams**

2 eggs

1 cup fresh mushrooms, quartered

2 slices of ham, evenly chopped

2 ounces feta (or other) cheese, crumbled

2 teaspoons vegetable oil or butter

½ bagel

Sauté mushrooms in a pan with butter or oil until mushrooms are tender. Remove from pan. Heat vegetable oil or butter in a pan at medium-high heat. Whisk eggs in a small bowl and pour them into the pan. Lift eggs at their edges with a spatula and tip the pan to make sure the egg mixture is cooked. Place mushrooms and ham over the eggs and cover with cheese. Turn the heat down to medium. Use your spatula to fold the omelet in half. Cook for 2-3 more minutes. Slide the omelet onto a plate. While omelet is cooking, toast bagel and butter.

NOTE: Serve alone or with up to 2 slices bacon or sausage. Remember to eat the bagel slowly and chew well.

Lunch: Miso Chicken Stew — Serves 6 — FP 8 grams

  1 pound boneless chicken thighs, chopped

  2 heads baby bok choy, chopped

  1 medium head broccoli, chopped

  4 large mushrooms, chopped

  1 small carrot, chopped

  ½ medium sweet onion, chopped

  2 green onion stems, finely chopped

  1 block tofu, cut in 1-inch cubes

  2 tablespoons vegetable oil

  8 tablespoons miso paste

  2 teaspoons fish bonito flakes

  Salt and pepper

Sauté chicken, onion and carrot together with a pinch of salt in one tablespoon vegetable oil with pepper on medium heat. Boil 6 cups water in a large pan. Add bonito flakes and chicken mixture and set to medium heat (to finish cooking carrots). Sauté broccoli in 2 teaspoons vegetable oil on medium high heat for about two minutes. Add bok choy and mushrooms and continue to sauté.

Add rest of vegetables and uncooked tofu into to stew pot with chicken veggie mix. Bring to a boil and reduce to simmer. Remove one cup of broth and dissolve miso into broth. Return to stew and mix well. Serve with sticky rice with chopped green onions sprinkled over the top. Some people like to add a little red pepper. We use S&B Hot Pepper Mix, but regular cayenne pepper works well too. Refrigerate leftovers for great lunches and appetizers.

Asian Sticky Rice — Serves 5

    1 cup rice

    1 cup water

Prepare sticky rice in advance. Rinse rice with cold water three to four times or until water runs clear. Mix rice with water and soak for 10 minutes prior to cooking in a rice cooker. Turn on the rice cooker. Don't open the lid for approximately 25 minutes. Let the rice sit for another 10 minutes. Fluff rice prior to serving.

Miso paste and bonito flakes are available in Asian markets and some grocery stores that carry Asian foods.

Snack: Kettle Corn Style Popcorn — Serves 2 — FP 5 grams

Follow the microwave directions to prepare popcorn. Add one tablespoon melted butter and mix in one tablespoon Splenda. Limit to ½ bag per person.

Dinner: Seared Tuna - Serves 2

    1 pound tuna steak (must be fresh!)

    2 tablespoons vegetable oil

    2 green onions, finely chopped

    4 sheets nori (edible seaweed)

    ¼ cup soy sauce

    2 teaspoons wasabi

    ½ pound tofu

    Cucumber salad (recipe below)

    Asian sticky rice (recipe below)

Pan-sear tuna in a very hot pan with a small amount of vegetable oil, cooking it for about 90 seconds on each side and searing the sides of the fish briefly as well by holding the fish on each of its sides. While the fish is cooking, prepare a large bowl of ice water with plenty of ice. Remove the tuna steaks from the heat while still red in the center, and plunge the tuna into ice water for five minutes to chill. Slice the seared tuna into thin 2 inch sashimi sized slices (about 1 ½ inches long) with a very sharp knife. Place fish on a chilled serving dish. Sprinkle uncooked, chopped green onions over the top.

Cut block of tofu into 1/3-inch thick slices and sauté with vegetable oil until both sides are brown. Top with soy sauce and uncooked, chopped green onions. Serve the tuna with tofu, cucumber salad and sticky rice along with soy sauce and wasabi for dipping the tuna. You can also wrap tuna pieces in nori (tear sheets in half or into quarters) and dip in soy sauce mixed with wasabi.

Asian Sticky Rice — Serves 5

1 cup rice

1 cup water

Prepare sticky rice in advance. Rinse rice with cold water three to four times or until water runs clear. Mix rice with water and soak for 10 minutes prior to cooking in a rice cooker. Turn on the rice cooker. Don't open the lid for approximately 25 minutes. Let the rice sit for another 10 minutes. Fluff rice prior to serving.

Cucumber and Seaweed Salad — Serves 2

½ English (or European) cucumber

¼ cup wakame (edible seaweed)

3 tablespoons vegetable oil

3 tablespoons rice vinegar

3 tablespoons soy sauce

1 teaspoon ginger, chopped

1 teaspoon Splenda

½ teaspoon cayenne pepper

Slice one half of the cucumber lengthwise to produce thin strips approximately two inches long. (These should look like matchsticks.) Rehydrate the wakame by adding ½ cup cold water. Let the seaweed sit for a few minutes before draining. Mix the cucumber strips with rehydrated wakame.

For dressing, mix three tablespoons each of vegetable oil, rice vinegar and soy sauce with 1 teaspoon chopped ginger, 1 teaspoon Splenda and a dash of cayenne pepper. Dress the salad just before serving.

Nori (edible sheets of dry seaweed) and wakame (dried shredded seaweed) are available at Asian grocery stores and some grocery stores that carry Asian foods.

Dessert: Key Lime Pie — Serves 1 — FP 5 grams

Serve a leftover piece of pie with whipped cream. Refer to recipe on day 9.

DAY 13 — Daily FP 29 grams

Breakfast: Smoked Salmon with Capers — Serves 2 — FP 4 grams

½ pound smoked salmon

½ ripe tomato, chopped

¼ sweet or red onion

1 tablespoon capers

2 tablespoon balsamic or white wine vinegar

Salt and pepper

If not pre-cut, slice the chilled salmon into thin strips and place onto a plate.

Cover with chopped tomato, onion, capers and balsamic or white wine vinegar. Add salt and pepper to taste and serve chilled.

Lunch: Greek Salad with Grilled Chicken — Serves 2 — FP 8 grams

- ½ head of lettuce

- ½ pound chicken breast

- ½ tomato, cut in wedges

- ¼ sweet onion

- 2 artichoke hearts in oil

- ¼ European (or regular) cucumber

- 6 black olives

- ½ cup feta cheese

- 2 tablespoons olive oil

- 2 tablespoons balsamic vinegar

Grill chicken breast or sauté with a small amount of vegetable oil, salt and pepper.

Mix vegetables with olive oil and vinegar. Top with feta cheese, chicken cut in strips and Greek dressing (recipe below). Serve

Greek Dressing — Serves 4

- ¾ cup extra virgin olive oil

- ¼ cup white vinegar

- 2 tablespoons lemon juice

- 1 garlic clove, minced

1 tablespoon dried oregano

1 tablespoon dried basil

1 pinch salt and pepper

Mix the olive oil, vinegar and lemon juice in a jar. Add the garlic, oregano, basil, and salt and pepper.

Snack: **Fruit Mix with Dates and Nuts — Serves 6 — FP 4 grams**

½ cup dates, sliced in half the long way

½ cup walnuts

1 cup strawberries, halved

½ cup pineapple, cubed

½ cup peaches, sliced in wedges

Mix nuts, fruit and dates and serve.

Dinner: **Steak Kabobs and Jasmine Rice — Serves 4 — FP 7 grams**

2 pounds steak, cut into 1 inch cubes

1 green bell pepper, cut into 1 inch squares

1 red pepper, cut into 1 inch squares

1 large onion, cut into 1 inch squares

6 large mushrooms, whole with stems cut flush

1/3 cup olive oil

1/3 cup soy sauce

½ lemon

½ cup fresh or 1 tablespoon dried basil, chopped

2 cloves garlic, minced and chopped

1 cup jasmine rice

1 ½ cups water

Prepare a marinade by combining olive oil, soy sauce, lemon juice, basil, garlic, and salt and pepper. Marinate the meat using a large zip-lock freezer bag. Refrigerate it for at least several hours, for as long as overnight. Just before cooking, add the peppers, onions and mushrooms to the bag and shake until coated. Slide the vegetable and steak pieces onto skewers. Add more salt and pepper if needed. Place skewers on a hot grill for about 4 to 6 minutes, turning them frequently and being sure not to overcook the meat.

Before grilling kabobs, combine rice with water in a medium saucepan (if using a rice cooker, use 1 ¾ cups water) and stir. Bring to boil uncovered on high heat. Reduce heat and simmer covered for 15 minutes. Don't remove the cover while cooking. Remove from heat and let stand covered for 5-7 minutes. Fluff with spatula before serving.

Lay skewers over jasmine rice and serve.

Note: If symptoms are gone, serve up to ¾ cup rice. If symptoms persist, limit rice to ½ cup servings.

Dessert: Ice Cream or Soy Creamy Frozen Dessert — Serves 1 — FP 6 grams

½ cup lactose-free Breyers ice cream (can increase to ¾

cup if symptoms are gone).

Serve the ice cream adding a few nuts and berries if desired. Alternatively, serve the same amount of Trader Joe's Soy Creamy Frozen Dessert. No other substitutions.

DAY 14 — Daily FP 47 Grams

Breakfast: White Toast with Cheese, Berries and Light Cream —

Serves 1 — FP 9 grams

>   1 slice white sandwich bread
>
>   2 slices cheddar (or other) cheese
>
>   2 teaspoons butter
>
>   ½ cup blackberries
>
>   ½ cup light cream
>
>   2 teaspoons Splenda

Toast bread, spread with butter and serve with sliced cheese and berries with cream sweetened with Splenda.

Eat the toast slowly and chew it well. Only have one slice. If this meal gives you heartburn, skip the toast for now. As your symptoms abate, you may be able to add it back. Try the toast again in one week.

Lunch: Sautéed Tofu and Veggies - Serves 2 — FP 8 grams

>   1 block tofu (14 ounces), diced
>
>   4 heads bok choy, chopped
>
>   3 green onions, finely chopped
>
>   1 tablespoon soy sauce
>
>   3 tablespoons vegetable oil
>
>   2 tablespoons oyster sauce

Add tofu to 1 tablespoon vegetable oil, salt and pepper, soy sauce and minced garlic in a pan. Sauté on medium to high heat for three to five minutes. Set aside. In the same pan, add 1 tablespoon vegetable oil and sauté the ground beef until browned. Mix ground beef with tofu and green onions. Add 1 tablespoon oyster sauce and 1 teaspoon soy sauce and mix and sauté for one or two more minutes.

Sauté bok choy in one tablespoon of oil. After two minutes, add a pinch of salt, 1 tablespoon oyster sauce and 1 teaspoon soy sauce and 2 to 3 tablespoons of water. Cover and simmer for another minute. The stalks should be tender and the leaves wilted. Be careful not to overcook. Serve with the tofu and ground beef.

Note: Oyster sauce is available in the Asian aisle of most grocery stores.

Snack: Spiced Nut Mix — Serves 1 — FP 14 grams

Refer to Day 3 Recipe

Limit to 3 Ounce daily Serving

Dinner: Lemon Chicken — Serves 2 — FP 10 grams

1 pound chicken breast, cut in strips

2 artichokes hearts (canned in water)

4 medium mushrooms

¼ cup white wine

1 ¼ teaspoon chicken bouillon powder

½ lemon

1 tablespoon capers

1 ½ tablespoon butter

1 tablespoon olive oil

1 clove garlic, sliced

Pepper

Marinate chicken with lemon juice, bouillon powder and pepper for 30 minutes refrigerated. Sauté garlic with butter and olive oil. Add chicken and sauté until almost cooked. Add artichokes, mushrooms and capers and sauté together. Turn the heat to high and add white wine. Continue to cook until wine evaporates. Serve with squash fries.

Squash Fries — Serves 5

> 1 small butternut squash, peeled and cut like French fries
>
> 2 tablespoons vegetable oil
>
> 2 tablespoons butter, melted
>
> Salt and pepper

Bake squash fries at 425 degrees on a non-stick oil-coated baking pan for about 45 minutes. Turn frequently to allow moisture to dissipate and squash to brown. Add salt and pepper and serve.

***Dessert*: Fruit Medley — Serves 5 — FP 6 grams**

> 1 cup watermelon, cubed
>
> 1 cup cantaloupe, cubed
>
> 1 cup strawberries, halved
>
> ½ cup pineapple, cubed
>
> ½ cup peaches, sliced in wedges
>
> ½ cup blueberries
>
> 1 lemon, cut in half

Wash and cut up fruit and combine in large bowl. Squeeze the juice of two lemon halves over the fruit salad, straining out any seeds. Serve chilled with or without whipped cream.

Note: Limit to a half cup serving if still having symptoms, otherwise, limit to a cup.

Whipped Cream — Serves 2

> 1 cup heavy cream, chilled

3 tablespoons Splenda

1 teaspoon vanilla extract

In a large mixing bowl, combine chilled cream, Splenda and vanilla extract. Set bowl inside a larger bowl filled with crushed ice. (This keeps the cream chilled.) Whip the cream with an electric mixer until light and fluffy.

Appendix B: Fermentation Potential Tables

Table 1 - Fermentation potential for *"Beans and Legumes"*

Beans and Legumes	Serving Size (oz)	Serving Size (grams)	Glycemic Index	Net Carbs per Serving (grams)	Fiber per Serving (grams)	Ferm. Potential (grams)	Relative Symptom Risk
Soy beans	5.3	150	20	6	6	11	Moderate
Peas, green	5.3	150	22	9	4	11	Moderate
Romano beans	5.3	150	46	18	3	12	Moderate
Mung bean	5.3	150	31	17	1	13	Moderate
Baked beans	5.3	150	48	15	6	14	Moderate
Split peas, yellow	5.3	150	32	19	12	25	High
Lentils	5.3	150	22	18	12	26	High
Butter beans	5.3	150	28	20	6	20	High
Brown beans	5.3	150	38	25	13	29	High
Pinto beans	5.3	150	39	26	13	29	High
Black beans	5.3	150	30	23	13	29	High
Kidney beans	5.3	150	23	25	11	31	High
Blackeyed beans	5.3	150	33	30	10	30	High
Lima beans	5.3	150	32	30	9	29	High
Chickpeas	5.3	150	31	30	6	27	High
Navy beans	5.3	150	30	30	16	37	High

Table 2 - Fermentation potential for *"Soups"*

Soups	Serving Size (oz)	Serving Size (grams)	Glycemic Index	Net Carbs per Serving (grams)	Fiber per Serving (grams)	Ferm. Potential (grams)	Relative Symptom Risk
*Miso Soup	8.8	250	50	2	2	2	Low
*Chicken Soup (no noodles)	8.8	250	50	2	1	2	Low
Black Bean soup	8.8	250	64	27	4	14	Moderate
Tomato soup	8.8	250	38	17	2	13	Moderate
Split Pea Soup	8.8	250	60	27	5	16	High
Minestrone Soup	8.8	250	39	18	6	17	High
Lentil Soup	8.8	250	44	21	12	24	High

* Glycemic index not available. An estimated GI of 50 was used.

Also note that you can estimate the FP of other soups by checking the FP or the ingredients. For instance, you can make a chicken soup without noodles but with lots of vegetables that will have a very low FP. Also check out the low FP clam chowder recipe in the recipe section.

Table 3 - Fermentation potential for *"Cookies and Crackers"*

Cookies and Crackers	Serving Size (oz)	Serving Size (grams)	Glycemic Index	Net Carbs per Serving (grams)	Fiber per Serving (grams)	Ferm. Potential (grams)	Relative Symptom Risk
Rice crackers	1	28	91	22	0	2	Low
Puffed rice cakes	1	28	82	24	0	5	Low
Water crackers	1	28	78	20	1	5	Low
Vanilla wafers	1	28	77	20	1	5	Low
Soda crackers (Saltines)	1	28	74	21	1	6	Low
Breton wheat crackers	1	28	67	16	1	6	Low
Graham crackers	1	28	71	20	1	7	Low
Shortbread cookies	1	28	64	18	0	7	Low
Oatmeal cookies	1	28	55	16	1	8	Moderate
Stoned Wheat Thins	1	28	67	19	2	8	Moderate
Rice cakes, (high-amylose rice)	1	28	61	24	1	11	Moderate
Rye crisp bread	1	28	63	18	6	13	Moderate

Note: Limit the quantity of flour-based snacks (especially wheat), eat slowly and chew well.

160

Table 4 - Fermentation potential for *"Breads"*

Breads	Serving Size (oz)	Serving Size (grams)	Glycemic Index	Net Carbs per Serving (grams)	Fiber per Serving (grams)	Ferm. Potential (grams)	Relative Symptom Risk
Baguette, white, plain	1.1	30	95	15	1	1	Low
Middle Eastern flatbread	1.1	30	97	16	1	1	Low
Rice bread, low-amylose rice	1.1	30	72	12	0	3	Low
Wonder™, white bread	1.1	30	80	15	1	4	Low
Gluten-free white bread	1.1	30	80	15	1	4	Low
English Muffin™	1.1	30	77	14	1	4	Low
White flour bread	1.1	30	70	14	1	5	Low
White wheat flour bread	1.1	30	73	15	1	5	Low
Kaiser rolls	1.1	30	73	16	1	6	Low
Whole meal flour bread	1.1	30	73	14	2	6	Low
Light rye bread	1.1	30	68	14	2	6	Low
Rice bread, high-amylose rice	1.1	30	61	12	2	7	Low
Muesli bread	1.1	30	54	12	2	8	Moderate
Healthy Choice™ Whole Grain Bread	1.1	30	62	14	2	8	Moderate
Wheat flour flatbread	1.1	30	66	16	2	8	Moderate

Breads	Serving Size (oz)	Serving Size (grams)	Glycemic Index	Net Carbs per Serving (grams)	Fiber per Serving (grams)	Ferm. Potential (grams)	Relative Symptom Risk
Pita bread, white	1.1	30	57	17	1	8	Moderate
100% Whole Grain™ bread	1.1	30	51	13	2	8	Moderate
Healthy Choice™ Hearty 7 Grain Bread	1.1	30	55	14	2	9	Moderate
Whole meal barley flour bread	1.1	30	70	20	3	9	Moderate
Pumpernickel	1.1	30	41	12	2	9	Moderate
Bagel, white	2.5	70	72	35	1	11	Moderate
Coarse wheat kernel bread	1.1	30	52	20	4	13	Moderate
Corn tortilla	1.8	50	52	24	2	13	Moderate
Coarse rye kernel bread	1.1	30	41	12	7	14	Moderate
Wheat tortilla	1.8	50	30	26	0	18	High

Note: Limit the quantity of bread, eat slowly and chew well. People who are sensitive to gluten should not consume bread made from wheat, rye or barley.

Table 5 - Fermentation potential for *"Cakes, Pastry and Muffins"*

Cakes, Pastry & Muffins	Serving Size (oz)	Serving Size (grams)	Glycemic Index	Net Carbs per Serving (grams)	Fiber per Serving (grams)	Ferm. Potential (grams)	Relative Symptom Risk
Corn muffin, low-amylose	2	57	102	29	2	1	Low
Scones, plain	2	57	92	18	0	2	Low
Pancakes, buckwheat, gluten-free,	2	57	102	16	5	5	Low
Waffles	2	57	76	21	1	6	Low
Doughnut	2	57	76	28	1	8	Moderate
Crumpet	2	57	69	22	1	8	Moderate
Croissant	2	57	67	26	2	10	Moderate
Apple muffin, made without sugar	2	57	48	18	1	10	Moderate
Cupcake, strawberry-iced	2	57	73	39	0	11	Moderate
Pastry	2	57	59	26	1	12	Moderate
Angel food cake	2	57	67	33	1	12	Moderate
Bran muffin	2	57	60	24	3	12	Moderate
Pop Tarts™, Double Chocolate (Kellogg's)	2	57	70	41	1	13	Moderate
Flan cake	2	57	65	39	0	14	Moderate
Pound cake	2	57	54	30	0	14	Moderate

Cakes, Pastry & Muffins	Serving Size (oz)	Serving Size (grams)	Glycemic Index	Net Carbs per Serving (grams)	Fiber per Serving (grams)	Ferm. Potential (grams)	Relative Symptom Risk
Pancakes, prepared from mix	2	57	67	41	1	14	Moderate
Oatmeal muffin	2	57	69	40	2	15	Moderate
Banana cake	2	57	47	27	1	15	Moderate
Chocolate butterscotch muffins	2	57	53	32	1	16	High
Apple muffin	2	57	44	28	1	16	High
Vanilla cake	2	57	42	30	0	18	High
Sponge cake, plain	2	57	46	33	0	18	High
Chocolate cake	2	57	38	27	2	18	High
Blueberry muffin	2	57	59	59	1	25	High

Note: Caution, some pancake mixes may have a lower glycemic index and hence higher Fermentative Potential.

In general, be careful with baked goods and anything made with wheat based flours. Focus on products made from low amylose rice and other low amylose gluten free products and, of course, eat slowly and chew well.

Table 6 - Fermentation potential for *"Cereals"*

Cereals	Serving Size (oz)	Serving Size (grams)	Glycemic Index	Net Carbs per Serving (grams)	Fiber per Serving (grams)	Ferm. Potential (grams)	Relative Symptom Risk
Cornflakes™ (Kellogg's)	1.1	30	92	26	1	3	Low
Rice Chex™ (Nabisco)	1.1	30	89	26	0	3	Low
Crispix™ (Kellogg's)	1.1	30	87	25	0	4	Low
Rice Krispies™ (Kellogg's)	1.1	30	82	26	0	5	Low
Corn Chex™ (Nabisco)	1.1	30	83	25	1	5	Low
Shredded Wheat™ (Nabisco)	1.1	30	83	20	4	7	Low
Special K™ (Kellogg's)	1.1	30	69	21	1	7	Low
Oat bran, raw	1.1	30	59	15	2	8	Moderate
Puffed Wheat (Quaker Oats)	1.1	30	67	20	1	8	Moderate
Cheerios™ (General Mills Inc)	1.1	30	74	20	3	8	Moderate
Golden Grahams™ (General Mills)	1.1	30	71	25	1	8	Moderate
*Cream of Wheat™, Instant (Nabisco)	8.8	250	74	30	1	9	Moderate
Grapenuts™ (Kraft Foods)	1.1	30	75	22	3	9	Moderate
Quick Oats (Quaker Oats Co)	1.1	30	65	14	4	9	Moderate
Oatmeal	1.1	30	54	20	0	10	Moderate

Cereals	Serving Size (oz)	Serving Size (grams)	Glycemic Index	Net Carbs per Serving (grams)	Fiber per Serving (grams)	Ferm. Potential (grams)	Relative Symptom Risk
Bran Flakes™ (Kellogg's)	1.1	30	74	18	5	10	Moderate
Raisin Bran™ (Kellogg's)	1.1	30	61	19	3	10	Moderate
Muesli, NS8	1.1	30	66	24	2	10	Moderate
Creamed porridge	1.1	30	59	23	1	10	Moderate
Life™ (Quaker Oats)	1.1	30	66	25	2	10	Moderate
Froot Loops™ (Kellogg's)	1.1	30	69	26	3	11	Moderate
Bran Chex™ Nabisco	1.1	30	58	19	4	12	Moderate
Hot cereal, apple & cinnamon (Con Agra)	1.1	30	37	22	1	15	High
All-Bran™ (Kellogg's)	1.1	30	38	23	9	23	High

Note: Caution, soy milk or lactose free milk is recommended for lower FP cereal preparation.

Also, limit wheat-based products, eat slowly and chew well.

Table 7 - Fermentation potential for *"Pasta"*

Pasta	Serving Size (oz)	Serving Size (grams)	Glycemic Index	Net Carbs per Serving (grams)	Fiber per Serving (grams)	Ferm. Potential (grams)	Relative Symptom Risk
Rice pasta, brown	6	170	92	36	2	5	Low
Tortellini, cheese	6	170	50	20	2	12	Moderate
*Rice noodles, (Thailand)	6	170	61	37	2	16	High
Rice vermicelli	6	170	58	37	1	17	High
Udon noodles	6	170	62	45	1	18	High
Macaroni and Cheese	6	170	64	48	1	18	High
Gluten-free pasta	6	170	54	40	1	20	High
Ravioli, meat filled	6	170	39	36	1	23	High
Mung bean noodles	6	170	39	43	1	27	High
Spaghetti	6	170	44	45	3	28	High
Macaroni, plain	6	170	45	46	3	28	High
Fettuccini	6	170	32	43	2	31	High

Most types of pasta should be avoided or significantly limited due to their high FP values.

Table 8 - Fermentation potential for "Rice and Potatoes"

Rice & Potatoes	Serving Size (oz)	Serving Size (grams)	Glycemic Index	Net Carbs per Serving (grams)	Fiber per Serving (grams)	Ferm. Potential (grams)	Relative Symptom Risk
Jasmine Rice	5.3	150	109	42	0	-3	Low
Potato, Desiree	5.3	150	101	17	2	2	Low
Glutinous short grain rice, white	5.3	150	98	32	2	3	Low
Potato, Pontiac	5.3	150	88	18	2	4	Low
Potato, Sebago	5.3	150	87	17	2	4	Low
Pelde rice, white	5.3	150	93	43	2	5	Low
Instant rice, white	5.3	150	87	42	1	6	Low
Potato, Russet	5.3	150	85	30	2	7	Low
Waxy rice (0-2% amylose)	5.3	150	88	43	2	7	Low
Calrose brown rice	5.3	150	87	38	3	8	Moderate
Calrose rice, white, medium grain	5.3	150	83	43	1	9	Moderate
Potato, Prince Edward Island	5.3	150	63	18	2	9	Moderate
French fries, frozen	5.3	150	75	29	4	11	Moderate
Pelde brown rice	5.3	150	76	38	3	12	Moderate
Millet	5.3	150	71	36	2	12	Moderate
Salted rice ball	5.3	150	80	52	2	12	Moderate

Rice & Potatoes	Serving Size (oz)	Serving Size (grams)	Glycemic Index	Net Carbs per Serving (grams)	Fiber per Serving (grams)	Ferm. Potential (grams)	Relative Symptom Risk
Potato, Ontario	5.3	150	58	27	2	13	Moderate
Roasted rice ball	5.3	150	77	54	2	14	Moderate
Doongara brown rice, high amylose	5.3	150	66	37	3	15	High
Basmati rice, high amylose, white	5.3	150	58	38	1	17	High
Arborio, risotto rice	5.3	150	69	53	1	18	High
Brown rice	5.3	150	50	33	3	19	High
Long grain (high amylose) rice	5.3	150	55	40	1	19	High
Converted, white rice, Uncle Ben's®	5.3	150	45	36	0	20	High
Sweet potato	5.3	150	48	34	4	21	High
Potato dumplings (with white flour)	5.3	150	52	45	2	24	High
Bangladeshi rice variety (28% amylose)	5.3	150	37	39	1	26	High

Table 9 - Fermentation potential for *"Vegetables"*

Vegetables	Serving Size (oz)	Serving Size (grams)	Glycemic Index	Net Carbs per Serving (grams)	Fiber per Serving (grams)	Ferm. Potential (grams)	Relative Symptom Risk
Chili, green	0.3	7	50	1	0	1	Low
Bok choy	2.8	80	50	0	1	1	Low
Lettuce	2.8	80	50	1	1	2	Low
Mixed greens	2.8	80	50	1	1	2	Low
Alfalfa sprouts	2.8	80	50	0	1	2	Low
Celery	2.8	80	50	1	1	2	Low
Arugula	2.8	80	50	0	2	2	Low
Pumpkin	2.8	80	75	4	1	2	Low
Cucumber	2.8	80	50	3	1	2	Low
Bamboo shoots	2.8	80	50	2	1	2	Low
Summer squash	2.8	80	50	3	1	2	Low
Radishes	2.8	80	50	2	1	2	Low
Zucchini	2.8	80	50	3	1	2	Low
Pepper, red, green	2.8	80	50	3	2	3	Low
Asparagus	2.8	80	50	2	2	3	Low
Mushrooms	2.8	80	50	3	1	3	Low

Vegetables	Serving Size (oz)	Serving Size (grams)	Glycemic Index	Net Carbs per Serving (grams)	Fiber per Serving (grams)	Ferm. Potential (grams)	Relative Symptom Risk
Rutabaga	**2.8**	**80**	**72**	**5**	**1**	**3**	Low
Chard	2.8	80	50	2	2	3	Low
Spinach	2.8	80	50	2	2	3	Low
Hearts of palm	2.8	80	50	2	2	3	Low
Tomatoes	2.8	80	50	4	1	3	Low
Cabbage, green, red	2.8	80	50	2	2	3	Low
Endive	2.8	80	50	1	3	3	Low
Rhubarb	2.8	80	50	3	2	3	Low
Cauliflower	2.8	80	50	3	2	3	Low
Daikon	2.8	80	50	3	2	3	Low
Parsnips	**2.8**	**80**	**97**	**12**	**3**	**3**	Low
Fennel	2.8	80	50	4	1	3	Low
Broccoli	2.8	80	50	2	3	4	Low
Eggplant	2.8	80	50	2	3	4	Low
Okra	2.8	80	50	4	2	4	Low
Turnips	2.8	80	50	5	2	4	Low
Artichoke	2.8	80	50	6	1	4	Low

Vegetables	Serving Size (oz)	Serving Size (grams)	Glycemic Index	Net Carbs per Serving (grams)	Fiber per Serving (grams)	Ferm. Potential (grams)	Relative Symptom Risk
Onion	2.8	80	50	6	1	4	Low
Tomato Sauce	4.0	112	50	8	1	5	Low
Beans, green	2.8	80	50	4	3	5	Low
Brussels sprouts	2.8	80	50	5	2	5	Low
Beans, wax	2.8	80	50	4	3	5	Low
Fennel	2.8	80	50	4	3	5	Low
Carrots	2.8	80	49	5	2	5	Low
Acorn squash	2.8	80	50	7	1	5	Low
Collard greens	2.8	80	50	5	3	6	Low
Snow peas	2.8	80	50	6	3	6	Low
Kale	2.8	80	50	9	2	6	Low
Winter squash	5.3	80	50	8	2	6	Low
Butternut squash	5.3	80	50	11	1	7	Low
Edamame	5.3	80	50	5	4	7	Low
Avocado	5.3	80	50	1	5	6	Low
Peas	5.3	80	54	7	4	8	Moderate
Sweet corn	5.3	80	60	18	1	9	Moderate

172

Vegetables	Serving Size (oz)	Serving Size (grams)	Glycemic Index	Net Carbs per Serving (grams)	Fiber per Serving (grams)	Ferm. Potential (grams)	Relative Symptom Risk
Yam	5.3	**80**	**66**	**19**	3	9	Moderate
Plantain	5.3	**80**	**40**	**23**	2	16	High

* Non-starchy vegetables are difficult to test for GI as subjects would need to consume very large amounts of each test food. As a result, many have not been tested. In these cases, a conservative estimated GI value of 50 has been used in the calculation of fermentative potential.

Fermentative Potential calculations based on measured GIs are listed in **bold** font.

Non-starchy vegetables are generally low in carbohydrates and moderate in fiber so the FP would be low regardless of the glycemic index.

Table 10 - Fermentation potential for *"Fruits"*

Fruits	Serving Size (oz)	Serving Size (grams)	Glycemic Index	Net Carbs per Serving (grams)	Fiber per Serving (grams)	Ferm. Potential (grams)	Relative Symptom Risk
Watermelon, fresh	4.2	120	72	6	0	2	Low
*Lemon, juice	2.1	60	50	4	0	2	Low
*Lime, juice	2.1	60	50	5	0	3	Low
Cantaloupe, fresh	4.2	120	65	6	1	3	Low
Dates, dried	2.1	60	103	20	5	4	Low
Strawberries, fresh	4.2	120	40	3	2	4	Low
Pineapple, fresh	4.2	120	66	10	2	5	Low
Peach, fresh	4.2	120	56	8	2	5	Low
Lychee, fresh	4.2	120	79	20	1	5	Low
Apricots, fresh	4.2	120	57	9	2	6	Low
Pear, canned	4.2	120	44	11	2	8	Moderate
Papaya, fresh	4.2	120	60	15	2	8	Moderate
Fruit cocktail	4.2	120	55	16	1	8	Moderate
*Blackberries, fresh	4.2	120	40	5	6	9	Moderate
Kiwi, fresh	4.2	120	58	12	4	9	Moderate
Apricots, canned	4.2	120	64	19	2	9	Moderate

Fruits	Serving Size (oz)	Serving Size (grams)	Glycemic Index	Net Carbs per Serving (grams)	Fiber per Serving (grams)	Ferm. Potential (grams)	Relative Symptom Risk
*Blueberries, fresh	4.2	120	40	12	3	10	Moderate
Strawberry jam	1.1	30	51	20	0	10	Moderate
Peach, canned	4.2	120	52	18	2	10	Moderate
Grapefruit, raw	4.2	120	25	11	2	10	Moderate
Orange marmalade	1.1	30	48	20	0	11	Moderate
Grapes	4.2	120	43	17	1	11	Moderate
*Coconut, shredded, unsweetened	2.1	60	50	7	8	11	Moderate
*Raspberries, fresh	4.2	120	40	7	8	12	Moderate
Cherries, raw	4.2	120	22	12	2	12	Moderate
Mango	4.2	120	51	20	2	12	Moderate
Plum	4.2	120	24	14	2	12	Moderate
Pear, raw	4.2	120	33	13	4	12	Moderate
Apple	4.2	120	40	16	3	12	Moderate
Banana, ripe	4.2	120	51	25	3	15	High
Banana, under ripe	4.2	120	30	21	3	18	High
Raisins	2.1	60	64	44	2	18	High
Apricots, dried	2.1	60	30	27	4	23	High

Fruits	Serving Size (oz)	Serving Size (grams)	Glycemic Index	Net Carbs per Serving (grams)	Fiber per Serving (grams)	Ferm. Potential (grams)	Relative Symptom Risk
Prunes, dried	2.1	60	29	33	4	28	High

* The glycemic index for blueberries, raspberries and black berries has not been determined, but has been estimated based on GI value for strawberries. The glycemic index for shredded coconut, lime and lemon juice was estimated to be 50%.

Note: To lower the FP value, reduce the serving size. For instance, ½ cup of blueberries weighs 74 grams (less than the 120 g shown in table) which has an FP of 6 grams — considered to be low.

Table 11 - Fermentation potential for *"Dairy and Soy Products"*

Dairy & Soy Products	Serving Size (oz)	Serving Size (grams)	Glycemic Index	Net Carbs per Serving (grams)	Fiber per Serving (grams)	Ferm. Potential (grams)	Relative Symptom Risk
[3]Heavy cream	8.0	227	50	3	0	2	Low
[3]Light cream	8.0	227	50	4	0	2	Low
[4]Soy milk, unsweetened	8.0	227	50	2	1	2	Low
[5]Almond drink	8.0	227	50	2	1	2	Low
[2]Lactose-free ice cream (Breyers)	4.0	113	61	14	0	5	Low
Yogurt, plain	8.0	227	36	10	0	7	Low
[1]Milk, whole	8.0	227	27	11	0	8	Moderate
[1]Milk, skim	8.0	227	32	12	0	8	Moderate
[1]Milk, condensed, sweetened	8.0	227	61	25	0	10	Moderate
[1]Milk, chocolate,	1.0	28	42	18	1	11	Moderate
[1]Ice cream	4.0	113	61	29	0	11	Moderate
[2]Carb Smart ice cream (Breyers)	4.0	113	61	4	4	11	Moderate
Yogurt, low-fat. fruit, aspartame sweetened	8.0	227	14	15	0	13	Moderate

Dairy & Soy Products	Serving Size (oz)	Serving Size (grams)	Glycemic Index	Net Carbs per Serving (grams)	Fiber per Serving (grams)	Ferm. Potential (grams)	Relative Symptom Risk
Yogurt, low-fat, fruit, sugar sweetened	8.0	227	33	35	0	24	High

[1]Lactose containing products such as milk, condensed milk and ice cream, though not likely yogurt, would have higher fermentative potentials if their glycemic index was determined with people who are lactose intolerant. If these foods give you symptoms, add dietary supplement lactase enzyme or reduce or eliminate lactose-containing foods. You can be tested for lactose intolerance.

[2]The GI for Breyers lactose free ice cream and Breyers Carb Smart ice cream was estimated based on the GI for other ice cream brands (61). Also, note that Breyers Carb Smart ice cream contains 5 grams of sugar alcohols (not shown in table) that must be added to the total FP resulting in an FP of 11 grams per 4 ounce serving.

[3]The GI for heavy and light cream estimated based on the GI for lactose (46).

[4]The GI for soy milk was estimated based on tofu (20).

[5]The GI for almond drink was estimated (50).

Table 12 - Fermentation potential for *"Non-Dairy Beverages"*

Non-Dairy Beverages	Serving Size (oz)	Serving Size (grams)	Glycemic Index	Net Carbs per Serving (grams)	Fiber per Serving (grams)	Ferm. Potential (grams)	Relative Symptom Risk
Diet soda and other zero calorie diet drinks	8.8	250	NA	0	0	0	Low
Rum, whiskey, vodka, etc	1.5	44	NA	0	0	0	Low
*Beer, lite	12.0	336	50	3	0	2	Low
*Wine, dry white	6.6	187	50	3	0	2	Low
*Wine, dry red	6.6	187	50	4	0	2	Low
Lucozade® (glucose drink)	8.8	250	95	42	0	2	Low
Gatorade®	8.8	250	78	15	0	3	Low
Quik™, chocolate mix dissolved in water	8.8	250	53	7	1	4	Low
*Beer, non-lite	12.0	336	50	12	0	6	Low
Tomato juice, no added sugar	8.8	250	38	9	1	7	Low
Coca Cola®, sweetened	8.8	250	63	26	0	10	Moderate
Grapefruit juice, unsweetened	8.8	250	48	20	0	11	Moderate
Cranberry juice cocktail	8.8	250	68	36	0	12	Moderate
Orange juice	8.8	250	57	26	1	12	Moderate
Hot Chocolate	8.8	250	51	23	1	12	Moderate

Non-Dairy Beverages	Serving Size (oz)	Serving Size (grams)	Glycemic Index	Net Carbs per Serving (grams)	Fiber per Serving (grams)	Ferm. Potential (grams)	Relative Symptom Risk
Carrot juice	8.8	250	43	23	2	15	High
Apple juice, unsweetened	8.8	250	40	29	1	18	High
Pineapple juice, unsweetened	8.8	250	46	34	1	19	High

*Beer and wine have not been tested for the glycemic index. A conservative estimated GI of 50 has been used.

Note that unsweetened mixed drinks, light beer and dry red or white wine are the lowest FP choices. Even though non-lite beer has an FP of only 6 grams, this can add up quickly if you drink more than one.

Also, avoid sweetened wines, as the FP will be considerably higher.

Table 13 - Fermentation potential for *"Desserts, Snacks, Nuts and Seeds"*

Desserts, Snacks, Nuts & Seeds	Serving Size (oz)	Serving Size (grams)	Glycemic Index	Net Carbs per Serving (grams)	Fiber per Serving (grams)	Ferm. Potential (grams)	Relative Symptom Risk
Rice cracker	1.1	30	91	25	0	2	Low
[2]Lactose-free ice cream (Breyers)	4.0	113	61	7	0	3	Low
Popcorn	0.7	20	89	11	3	4	Low
Pretzels	1.1	30	83	20	1	4	Low
[1]Pecans	1.1	30	22	1	3	4	Low
[1]Walnuts	1.1	30	22	2	2	4	Low
Peanuts	1.1	30	7	2	2	5	Low
[1]Almonds	1.1	30	22	2	3	5	Low
[1]Almond meal	1.1	30	22	2	3	5	Low
Rice pudding	2.6	75	59	11	1	5	Low
Hummus (chickpea salad dip)	1.1	30	6	5	2	6	Low
Cashews	1.1	30	22	8	1	7	Low
Life Savers® candy (Nestlé)	1.1	30	70	30	0	9	Moderate
Corn chips	1.8	50	72	25	3	10	Moderate
Custard	3.5	100	43	17	0	10	Moderate
[3]Ice cream	4.0	113	61	30	0	12	Moderate

Desserts, Snacks, Nuts & Seeds	Serving Size (oz)	Serving Size (grams)	Glycemic Index	Net Carbs per Serving (grams)	Fiber per Serving (grams)	Ferm. Potential (grams)	Relative Symptom Risk
[1,3]Carb Smart ice cream (Breyers)	4.0	113	61	4	4	11	Moderate
Pop Tarts™, (Kellogg's)	1.8	50	70	35	1	11	Moderate
Pizza, cheese	3.5	100	60	27	2	12	Moderate
Snickers Bar® (Mars)	2.1	60	68	34	1	12	Moderate
M & M's®, peanut (Mars)	1.1	30	33	17	1	12	Moderate
Potato chips	1.8	50	51	24	2	13	Moderate
Skittles® (Mars)	1.8	50	70	45	0	14	Moderate
Milk chocolate	1.6	44	43	25	1	15	High
Mars Bar® (Mars)	2.1	60	62	40	1	16	High
Twix® Cookie Bar (Mars)	2.1	60	44	39	1	23	High

[1]Almonds, almond meal, pecans, walnuts and Carb Smart ice cream have not been assigned a GI value. The GI values were estimated based on similar foods.

[2]Breyers makes lactose free ice cream with 14 grams net carbs and no fiber per 1/2 cup. The GI was estimated based on the GI for other ice cream brands.

[3]Lactose-containing products such as milk, condensed milk and ice cream, and possibly yogurt, would have higher fermentative potentials if their glycemic index were determined in lactose intolerant people. If these foods give you symptoms, add dietary supplement lactase enzyme or reduce or eliminate lactose-containing foods. You can be tested for lactose intolerance.

Table 14 - Fermentation potential for *"Sweeteners"*

Sweeteners	Serving Size (oz)	Serving Size (grams)	Glycemic Index	Net Carbs per Serving (grams)	Fiber per Serving (grams)	Ferm. Potential (grams)	Relative Symptom Risk
Maltose	0.5	14	105	14	0	-1	Low
NutraSweet	0.5	14	NA	0	0	0	Low
Saccharin	0.5	14	NA	0	0	0	Low
Glucose	0.5	14	100	14	0	0	Low
[1]Splenda	0.5	14	*100	7	0	0	Low
Sucrose	0.5	14	59	14	0	6	Low
[2]Brown sugar	0.5	14	59	14	0	6	Low
Honey	0.5	14	55	14	0	6	Low
Lactose	0.5	14	48	14	0	7	Low
Fructose	0.5	14	20	14	0	11	Moderate

Note: The FP of glucose is zero by definition because glucose is completely absorbed. NutraSweet and saccharin have zero carbs and hence have a fermentative potential of zero. Lactose gives a relatively low FP but the GI was determined in volunteers that likely were not lactose intolerant. The effective FP for lactose intolerant people, if measured, would be much higher potentially approaching the NC value. Also, notice the extreme low GI/high FP for fructose, which is absorbed very poorly.

[1]Splenda has 14 grams of carbs per 1/2 ounce, but the carbs are in the form of maltodextrin, a partial breakdown product of starch. Maltodextrin is absorbed as efficiently as glucose; hence Splenda has an FP equal to zero.

183

[2]The glycemic index for brown sugar was estimated to be 59, the same as sucrose (table sugar).

Table 15 - Fermentation potential for *"Meat, Cheese, Tofu and Seafood"*

Meat, Cheese, Tofu & Seafood	Serving Size (oz)	Serving Size (grams)	Glycemic Index	Net Carbs per Serving (grams)	Fiber per Serving (grams)	Ferm. Potential (grams)	Relative Symptom Risk
Steak	6	170	NA	0	0	0	Low
Hamburg	6	170	NA	0	0	0	Low
Pork	6	170	NA	0	0	0	Low
Hotdog	6	170	NA	0	0	0	Low
Ham	6	170	NA	0	0	0	Low
Chicken	6	170	NA	0	0	0	Low
[1]Tofu	4.5	126	20	1	1	2	Low
Duck	6	170	NA	0	0	0	Low
Fish	6	170	NA	0	0	0	Low
Seafood	6	170	NA	0	0	0	Low
[2]Scallops	8	170	50	4	0	2	Low
Cold cuts	4	114	NA	0	0	0	Low
[3]Swiss Cheese	2	57	NA	0	0	0	Low
[3]Cheddar Cheese	2	57	NA	0	0	0	Low
[3]Mozzarella Cheese	2	57	48	1	0	1	Low
[3]American Cheese	2	57	48	4	0	2	Low

Meat, Cheese, Tofu & Seafood	Serving Size (oz)	Serving Size (grams)	Glycemic Index	Net Carbs per Serving (grams)	Fiber per Serving (grams)	Ferm. Potential (grams)	Relative Symptom Risk
[3]Cream cheese	2	57	48	3	0	1	Low
[3]Ricotta Cheese	2	57	48	2	0	1	Low

[1]Tofu has not been tested for the glycemic index - assume a glycemic index of 20 based on soy beans.

[2]Scallops have not been tested for the glycemic index - assume a glycemic index of 50%

[3]Most cheeses have low overall carb counts and hence were not assessed for glycemic index. The GI for lactose (48) was used to calculate the FP for cheeses. These foods have a Fermentative Potential [FP] close to zero. The symptom potential for these foods is therefore low. The lactose content (because cheese comes from milk) may be an issue for some lactose intolerant people. Limit cheeses, such as Ricotta, with the higher carbs counts if you are lactose intolerant or take lactase enzyme with cheese-containing meals.

Appendix C: Fast Tract Dietary Journal Template

Name: **Date:**

MEAL	DESCRIPTION	FP
Breakfast		
Snack		
Lunch		
Snack		
Dinner		
Snack		
	DAILY FP-TOTALS	

OBSERVED SYMPTOMS:

188

Name: **Date:**

MEAL	DESCRIPTION	FP
Breakfast		
Snack		
Lunch		
Snack		
Dinner		
Snack		
	DAILY FP-TOTALS	

OBSERVED SYMPTOMS:

189

Name: Date:

MEAL	DESCRIPTION	FP
Breakfast		
Snack		
Lunch		
Snack		
Dinner		
Snack		
	DAILY FP-TOTALS	

OBSERVED SYMPTOMS:

Name: **Date:**

MEAL	DESCRIPTION	FP
Breakfast		
Snack		
Lunch		
Snack		
Dinner		
Snack		
	DAILY FP-TOTALS	

OBSERVED SYMPTOMS:

191

Name: Date:

MEAL	DESCRIPTION	FP
Breakfast		
Snack		
Lunch		
Snack		
Dinner		
Snack		
	DAILY FP-TOTALS	

OBSERVED SYMPTOMS:

Name: **Date:**

MEAL	DESCRIPTION	FP
Breakfast		
Snack		
Lunch		
Snack		
Dinner		
Snack		
	DAILY FP-TOTALS	

OBSERVED SYMPTOMS:

Name: **Date:**

MEAL	DESCRIPTION	FP
Breakfast		
Snack		
Lunch		
Snack		
Dinner		
Snack		
	DAILY FP-TOTALS	

OBSERVED SYMPTOMS:

Index

digestive enzyme deficiency,
  58–59
gastric (stomach) acid
  reduction, 53–54
immune impairment, 54–55
intestinal epithelium damage,
  56–57
motility issues, 49–51

V
vagus nerve damage, 49–50
verbascose, 75
vitamin and mineral
  supplements, 21, 96–97

W
water, 21, 95
weighing foods, 103
wheat products, 104
whole-grain foods, 94

X
xylitol, 76

Y
yogurt, 52, 87–88, 177–178

Final Note

I founded the Digestive Health Institute to conduct research on digestive health conditions and identify and share holistic treatment approaches. The web site address is http://www.DigestiveHealthInstitute.org.

Fast Tract Digestion — Heartburn is one of a series of books on digestive illness involving SIBO and carbohydrate malabsorption. For the latest news on the book series check out the web site http://www.fasttractdigestion.com.

Thank you for reading *Fast Tract Digestion — Heartburn*. I hope you find this unique perspective on chronic acid reflux helpful, try some of the recipes, and most importantly; have noticed an improvement in your acid reflux symptoms.

If you found value in this book, please tell a friend or spread the word through social media.

References

Most of the references cited in this book can be found on the PubMed web site. In most cases only the abstract is available for free, but sometimes the entire article is available. The link to the website is http://www.ncbi.nlm.nih.gov/pubmed/.

Thanks!

End Notes

[1] Locke GR 3rd, Talley NJ, Fett SL, Zinsmeister AR, Melton LJ 3rd. Prevalence and clinical spectrum of gastroesophageal reflux: a population-based study in Olmsted County, Minnesota. Gastroenterology 1997; 112: 1448-1456.

[2] Hirschowitz BI, Worthington J, Mohnen J. Vitamin B12 deficiency in hypersecretors during long-term acid suppression with proton pump inhibitors. Aliment Pharmacol Ther. 2008. Jun 1;27(11):1110-21. Marcuard SP, Albernaz L, Khazanie PG. Omeprazole therapy causes malabsorption of cyanocobalamin (vitamin B12). Ann Intern Med. 1994 Feb 1;120(3):211-5. Patel TA, Abraham P, Ashar VJ, Bhatia SJ, Anklesaria PS. Gastric bacterial overgrowth accompanies profound acid suppression. Indian J Gastroenterol. 1995 Oct;14(4):134-6. Fried M, Siegrist H, Frei R, Froehlich F, Duroux P, Thorens J, Blum A, Bille J, Gonvers JJ, Gyr C. Duodenal bacterial overgrowth during treatment in outpatients with omeprazole. Gut 1994; 35:23-26. Shindo K, Machida M, Fukumura M, Koide K, Yamazaki R. Omeprazole induces altered bile acid metabolism. Gut. 1998 Feb;42(2):266-71. Theisen J, Nehra D, Citron D, Johansson J, Hagen JA, Crookes PF, DeMeester SR, Bremner CG, DeMeester TR, Peters JH. Suppression of gastric acid secretion in patients with gastroesophageal reflux disease results in gastric bacterial overgrowth and deconjugation of bile acids. J Gastrointest. Surg. 2000 Jan-Feb;4(1):50-4. Lombardo L, Foti M, Ruggia O, Chiecchio A. Increased incidence of small intestinal bacterial overgrowth during proton pump inhibitor therapy. Clin Gastroenterol Hepatol. 2010 Jun;8(6):504-8.

[3] Dial S, Delaney JA, Barkun AN, Suissa S. Use of gastric acid-suppressive agents and the risk of community-acquired *Clostridium difficile*-associated disease. JAMA. 2005 Dec 21;294(23):2989-95.

[4] Cadle RM, Mansouri MD, Logan N, Kudva DR, Musher DM. Association of proton-pump inhibitors with outcomes in Clostridium difficile colitis. Am J Health-Syst Pharm. 2007 Nov 15;64(22):2359-60.

[5] Laheij RJ, Sturkenboom MC, Hassing RJ, Dieleman J, Stricker BH, Jansen JB. Risk of community-acquired pneumonia and use of gastric acid-suppressive drugs. JAMA. 2004 Oct 27;292(16):1955-60.

[6] Canani RB, Cirillo P, Roggero P, Romano C, Malamisura B, Terrin G, et al. Therapy with gastric acidity inhibitors increases the risk of acute gastroenteritis and community-acquired pneumonia in children. Pediatrics 2006;117:e817-20.

[7] Yang YX, Lewis JD, Epstein S, Metz DC. Long-term proton pump inhibitor therapy and risk of hip fracture. JAMA. 2006 Dec 27;296(24):2947-53.

[8] Penagini R. Fat and gastro-oesophageal reflux disease. Eur J Gastroenterol Hepatol. 2000 Dec;12(12):1343-5.

[9] Pehl C, Waizenhoefer A, Wendl B, Schmidt T, Schepp W, Pfeiffer A. Effect of low and high fat meals on lower esophageal sphincter motility and gastroesophageal reflux in healthy subjects. Am J Gastroenterol. 1999 May;94(5):1192-6.

[10] *Heartburn Cured*. Robillard N. Self Health Publishing, 2005. ISBN 0-9766425-0-6. Available on Amazon.com.

[11] Booyens J, Louwrens CC, Katzeff IE. The role of unnatural dietary trans and cis unsaturated fatty acids in the epidemiology of coronary artery disease. Med Hypotheses 1988; 25:175-182. Grundy SM, Abate N, Chandalia M. Diet composition and the metabolic syndrome: what is the optimal fat intake? Am J Med. 2002 Dec 30; 113 Suppl 9B:25S-29S.

[12] United States Food and Drug Administration, September 8, 2004. FDA announces qualified health claims for omega-3 fatty acids. Press release.

[13] Rada V, Bartonová J, Vlková E. Specific growth rate of bifidobacteria cultured on different sugars. Folia Microbiol (Praha). 2002;47(5):477-80.

[14] Bouhnik Y, Alain S, Attar A, Flourié B, Raskine L, Sanson-Le Pors MJ, Rambaud JC. Bacterial populations contaminating the upper gut in patients with small intestinal bacterial overgrowth syndrome. Am J Gastroenterol. 1999 May;94(5):1327-31). Ghoshal U, Ghoshal UC, Ranjan P, Naik SR, Ayyagari A. Spectrum and antibiotic sensitivity of bacteria contaminating the upper gut in patients with malabsorption syndrome from the tropics. BMC Gastroenterol. 2003 May 24;3:9.

[15] Bouhnik Y, Alain S, Attar A, Flourié B, Raskine L, Sanson-Le Pors MJ, Rambaud JC. Bacterial populations contaminating the upper gut in patients with small intestinal bacterial overgrowth syndrome. Am J Gastroenterol. 1999 May;94(5):1327-31). Ghoshal U, Ghoshal UC, Ranjan P, Naik SR, Ayyagari A. Spectrum and antibiotic sensitivity of bacteria

contaminating the upper gut in patients with malabsorption syndrome from the tropics. BMC Gastroenterol. 2003 May 24;3:9.

[16] Dener IA, Demirci C. Explosion during diathermy gastrotomy in a patient with carcinoma of the antrum. Int J Clin Pract. 2003 Oct; 57(8):737-8. Bigard M-A, Gaucher P, Lassalle C. Fatal colonic explosion during colonoscopic polypectomy. Gastroenterology 1979; 77: 1307-1310.

[17] Yancy WS Jr, Provenzale D, Westman EC. Improvement of gastroesophageal reflux disease after initiation of a low-carbohydrate diet: five brief cased reports. Altern Ther health med. 2001. Nov-Dec; 7(6):120,116-119. Austin GL, Thiny MT, Westman EC, Yancy WS Jr, Shaheen NJ. A very low-carbohydrate diet improves gastroesophageal reflux and its symptoms. Dig Dis Sci. 2006 Aug;51(8):1307-12.

[18] Pennathur A, Tran A, Cioppi M, Fayad J, Sieren GL, Little AG. Erythromycin strengthens the defective lower esophageal sphincter in patients with gastroesophageal reflux disease. Am J Surg. 1994 Jan;167(1):169-173. Pehl C, Pfeiffer A, Wendl B, Stellwag B, Kaess H. Effect of erythromycin on postprandial gastroesophageal reflux in reflux esophagitis. Dis Esophagus. 1997 Jan;10(1):34-37.

[19] Mertens V, Blondeau K, Pauwels A, Farre R, Vanaudenaerde B, Vos R, Verleden G, Van Raemdonck DE, Dupont LJ, Sifrim D. Azithromycin reduces gastroesophageal reflux and aspiration in lung transplant recipients. Dig Dis Sci. 2009 May;54(5):972-9.

[20] Piche T, des Varannes SB, Sacher-Huvelin S, Holst JJ, Cuber JC, Galmiche JP. Colonic fermentation influences lower esophageal sphincter function in gastroesophageal reflux disease. Gastroenterology. 2003 Apr;124(4):894-902.

[21] Dodds WJ, Dent J, Hogan WK, Helm JF, Hauser R, Patel GK, Egide MS, Mechanisms of gastroesophageal reflux in patients with reflux esophagitis. N. Engl J Med. 1982. Dec 16;307(25):1547-52. Lin M, Triadafilopoulos G. Belching: dyspepsia or gastroesophageal reflux disease? Am J Gastroenterol. 2003 Oct;98(10):2139-45.

[22] Vakil N, Shaw M, Kirby R. Clinical effectiveness of laparoscopic fundoplication in a US community. Am J Med. 2003 Jan;114(1):1-5. Klaus A, Hinder RA, DeVault KR, Achem SR. Bowel dysfunction after laparoscopic anti reflux surgery: incidence, severity, and clinical course. Am J Med. 2003 Jan;114(1):6-9. Beldi G, Glättli A. Long-term

gastrointestinal symptoms after laparoscopic Nissen fundoplication. Surg Laparosc Endosc Percutan Tech. 2002 Oct;12(5):316-9.

23 Ledson MJ, Tran J, Walshaw MJ. Prevalence and mechanisms of gastro-oesophageal reflux in adult cystic fibrosis patients. J R Soc Med. 1998 Jan;91(1):7-9. Vic P, Tassin E, Turck D, Gottrand F, Launay V, Farriaux JP. Frequency of gastroesophageal reflux in infants and in young children with cystic fibrosis. Arch Pediatr. 1995 Aug;2(8):742-6. Fridge JL, Conrad C, Gerson L, Castillo RO, Cox K. Risk factors for small bowel bacterial overgrowth in cystic fibrosis. J Pediatr Gastroenterol Nutr. 2007 Feb;44(2):212-8.

24 Nastaskin I, Mehdikhani E, Conklin J, Park S, Pimentel M. Studying the overlap between IBS and GERD: a systematic review of the literature. Dig Dis Sci. 2006. Dec;51(12):2113-20.

25 Pimentel M, Chow EJ, Lin HC. Eradication of small intestinal bacterial overgrowth reduces symptoms of irritable bowel syndrome. Am J Gastroenterol. 2000;95:3503-6. Austin GL, Dalton CB, Hu Y, Morris CB, Hankins J, Weinland SR, Westman EC, Yancy WS Jr, Drossman DA. A very low-carbohydrate diet improves symptoms and quality of life in diarrhea-predominant irritable bowel syndrome. Clin Gastroenterol Hepatol. 2009 Jun;7(6):706-708. Majewski M, Reddymasu SC, Sostarich S, Foran P, McCallum RW. Efficacy of rifaximin, a non absorbed oral antibiotic, in the treatment of small intestinal bacterial overgrowth. Am J Med Sci. 2007 May;333(5):266-70. Pimentel M. Review of rifaximin as treatment for SIBO and IBS. Expert Opin Investig Drugs. 2009 Mar;18(3):349-58. Yang J, Lee HR, Low K, Chatterjee S, Pimentel M. Rifaximin versus other antibiotics in the primary treatment and retreatment of bacterial overgrowth in IBS. Dig Dis Sci. 2008 Jan;53(1):169-74.

26 Hagen J, Deitel M, Khanna RK, Ilves R. Gastroesophageal reflux in the massively obese. Int. Surg. 1987 Jan-Mar;72(1):1-3. Fisher BL, Pennathur A, Mutnick JL, Little AG. Obesity correlates with gastroesophageal reflux. Dig Dis Sci. 1999 Nov;44(11):2290-4. Austin GL, Thiny MT, Westman EC, Yancy WS Jr, Shaheen NJ. A very low-carbohydrate diet improves gastroesophageal reflux and its symptoms (Obese patients). Dig Dis Sci. 2006 Aug;51(8):1307-12.

27 Lombardo L, Foti M, Ruggia O, Chiecchio A. Increased incidence of small intestinal bacterial overgrowth during proton pump inhibitor therapy. Clin Gastroenterol Hepatol. 2010 Jun;8(6):504-8

[28] Pimentel M, Chow EJ, Lin HC. Eradication of small intestinal bacterial overgrowth reduces symptoms of irritable bowel syndrome. Am J Gastroenterol. 2000;95:3503-6.

[29] Pimental M. A New IBS Solution. Health Point Press. 2006.

[30] Rumessen JJ, Gudmand-Høyer E. Functional bowel disease: malabsorption and abdominal distress after ingestion of fructose, sorbitol, and fructose-sorbitol mixtures. Gastroenterology. 1988 Sep;95(3):694-700. Novillo A, Peralta D, Dima G, Besasso H, Soifer L. Frequency of bacterial overgrowth in patients with clinical lactose intolerance. Acta Gastroenterol Latinoam. 2010 Sep;40(3):221-4.

[31] Khoruts A, Dicksved J, Jansson JK, Sadowsky MJ. Changes in the composition of the human fecal microbiome after bacteriotherapy for recurrent Clostridium difficile-associated diarrhea. J Clin Gastroenterol. 2010 May-Jun;44(5):354-60. Bakken JS. Fecal bacteriotherapy for recurrent Clostridium difficile infection. Anaerobe. 2009 Dec;15(6):285-9. Dr. Johan S. Bakken. Personal communication on updated number of C diff cases treated with bacteriotherapy. February 2011.

[32] Borody TJ, Warren EF, Leis SM, Surace R, Ashman O, Siarakas S. Bacteriotherapy using fecal flora: toying with human motions. J Clin Gastroenterol. 2004 Jul;38(6):475-83.

[33] Grehan MJ, Borody TJ, Leis SM, Campbell J, Mitchell H, Wettstein A. Durable alteration of the colonic microbiota by the administration of donor fecal flora. J Clin Gastroenterol. 2010 Sep;44(8):551-61.

[34] Fossmark R, Johnsen G, Johanessen E, Waldum HL. Rebound acid hypersecretion after long-term inhibition of gastric acid secretion. Aliment Pharmacol Ther. 2005 Jan 15;21(2):149-54.

[35] Reimer C, Søndergaard B, Hilsted L, Bytzer P. Proton-pump inhibitor therapy induces acid-related symptoms in healthy volunteers after withdrawal of therapy. Gastroenterology. 2009 Jul;137(1):80-7.

[36] Patel TA, Abraham P, Ashar VJ, Bhatia SJ, Anklesaria PS. Gastric bacterial overgrowth accompanies profound acid suppression. Indian J Gastroenterol. 1995 Oct;14(4):134-6. Fried M, Siegrist H, Frei R, Froehlich F, Duroux P, Thorens J, Blum A, Bille J, Gonvers JJ, Gyr C. Duodenal bacterial overgrowth during treatment in outpatients with omeprazole. Gut 1994; 35:23-26. Shindo K, Machida M, Fukumura M, Koide K, Yamazaki R. Omeprazole induces altered bile acid metabolism. Gut. 1998

Feb;42(2):266-71. Theisen J, Nehra D, Citron D, Johansson J, Hagen JA, Crookes PF, DeMeester SR, Bremner CG, DeMeester TR, Peters JH. Suppression of gastric acid secretion in patients with gastroesophageal reflux disease results in gastric bacterial overgrowth and deconjugation of bile acids. J Gastrointest Surg. 2000 Jan-Feb;4(1):50-4. Lombardo L, Foti M, Ruggia O, Chiecchio A. Increased incidence of small intestinal bacterial overgrowth during proton pump inhibitor therapy. Clin Gastroenterol Hepatol. 2010 Jun;8(6):504-8.

[37] Lauritano EC, Bilotta AL, Gabrielli M, et al. Association between hypothyroidism and small intestinal bacterial overgrowth. J Clin Endocrinol Metab. 2007 Nov;92(11):4180-4.

[38] Pimentel M, Soffer EE, Chow EJ, et al. Lower frequency of MMC is found in IBS subjects with abnormal lactulose breath test, suggesting bacterial overgrowth. Dig Dis Sci, 2002;47:2639-2643.

[39] Ghoshal UC, Ghoshal U, Das K, Misra A. Utility of hydrogen breath tests in diagnosis of small intestinal bacterial overgrowth in malabsorption syndrome and its relationship with oro-cecal transit time. Indian J Gastroenterol. 2006 Jan-Feb;25(1):6-10.

[40] Lombardo L, Foti M, Ruggia O, Chiecchio A. Increased incidence of small intestinal bacterial overgrowth during proton pump inhibitor therapy. Clin Gastroenterol Hepatol. 2010 Jun;8(6):504-8.

[41] Lin, HC, Zaidel, O. Uninvited Guests: The Impact of Small Intestinal Bacterial Overgrowth on Nutritional Status. Nutrition Issues in Gastroenterology, Series #7. Practical Gastroenterology. Jul 2003. PP 27-34.

[42] Riepe SP, Goldstein J, Alpers DH. Effect of secreted Bacteroides proteases on human intestinal brush border hydrolases. J Clin Invest. 1980 Aug;66(2):314-22. Jonas A, Krishnan C, Forstner G. Pathogenesis of mucosal injury in the blind loop syndrome. Gastroenterology. 1978 Nov;75(5):791-5.

[43] Mishkin B, Yalovsky M, Mishkin S. Increased prevalence of lactose malabsorption in Crohn's disease patients at low risk for lactose malabsorption based on ethnic origin. Am J Gastroenterol. 1997 Jul;92(7):1148-53.

[44] Fisher BL, Pennathur A, Mutnick JL, Little AG. Obesity correlates with gastroesophageal reflux. Dig Dis Sci. 1999 Nov;44(11):2290-4. Teitelbaum

JE, Sinha P, Micale M, Yeung S, Jaeger J. Obesity is related to multiple functional abdominal diseases. J Pediatr. 2009 Mar;154(3):444-6.

[45] Delgado-Aros S, Locke GR 3rd, Camilleri M, Talley NJ, Fett S, Zinsmeister AR, Melton LJ 3rd. Obesity is associated with increased risk of gastrointestinal symptoms: a population-based study. Am J Gastroenterol. 2004 Sep;99(9):1801-6.

[46] Wynckel A, Jaisser F, Wong T, Drueke T, Chanard J. Intestinal Absorption of calcium from yogurt in lactase-deficient subjects. Reprod Nutr Dev. 1991; 31(4):411-8 and Kolars JC, Levitt MD, Aouji, Savaiano DA. Yogurt — an autodigesting source of lactose. N engl J Med 1984 Jan 5;310(1):1-3.

[47] Barrett JS, Irving PM, Shepherd SJ, Muir JG, Gibson PR. Comparison of the prevalence of fructose and lactose malabsorption across chronic intestinal disorders. Aliment Pharmacol Ther. 2009 Jul 1;30(2):165-74. Gibson PR, Newnham E, Barrett JS, Shepherd SJ, Muir JG. Review article: fructose malabsorption and the bigger picture. Aliment Pharmacol Ther. 2007 Feb 15;25(4):349-63.

[48] Helliwell PA, Richardson M, Affleck J, Kellett GL. Regulation of GLUT5, GLUT2 and intestinal brush-border fructose absorption by the extracellular signal-regulated kinase, p38 mitogen-activated kinase and phosphatidylinositol 3-kinase intracellular signaling pathways: implications for adaptation to diabetes. Biochem J. 2000 Aug 15;350 Pt 1:163-9.

[49] Shepherd SJ, Gibson PR. Fructose malabsorption and symptoms of irritable bowel syndrome: guidelines for effective dietary management. J Am Diet Assoc. 2006 Oct;106 (10):1631-9.

[50] Rumessen JJ, Gudmand-Høyer E. Absorption capacity of fructose in healthy adults. Comparison with sucrose and its constituent monosaccharides. Gut. 1986 Oct;27(10):1161-8.

[51] Anderson IH, Lavine AS, Levitt MD. Incomplete absorption of carbohydrate in all-purpose wheat flour. N Engl J Med. 1981 Apr 9;304(15):891-2. Levitt MD, Hirsh P, Fetzer CA, Sheahan M, Levine AS. H2 excretion after ingestion of complex carbohydrates. Gastroenterology. 1987 Feb;92(2):383-9.

[52] Stephen AM. Starch and dietary fibre: their physiological and epidemiological interrelationships. Can J Physiol Pharmacol. 1991 Jan;69(1):116-20.

[53] Hallfrisch J, Behall KM. Breath hydrogen and methane responses of men and women to breads made with white flour or whole wheat flours of different particle sizes. J Am Coll Nutr. 1999 Aug;18(4):296-302.

[54] Englyst HN, Trowell H, Southgate DA, Cummings JH. Dietary fiber and resistant starch. Am J Clin Nutr. 1987 Dec;46(6):873-4. Bird AR, Brown IL, Topping DL. Starches, resistant starches, the gut microflora and human health. Curr Issues Intest Microbiol. 2000 Mar;1(1):25-37.

[55] Bird AR, Brown IL, Topping DL. Starches, resistant starches, the gut microflora and human health. Curr Issues Intest Microbiol. 2000 Mar;1(1):25-37.

[56] Gidley MJ, Cooke D, Darke AH, Hoffmann RA, Russell AL, Greenwell P. Molecular order and structure in enzyme-resistant retrograded starch. Carbohydrate Polymers, 28(1)1995. 23-31.

[57] Macfarlane GT, Englyst HN. Starch utilization by the human large intestinal microflora. J Appl Bacteriol. 1986 Mar;60(3):195-201. Wang X, Conway PL, Brown IL, Evans AJ. In vitro utilization of amylopectin and high-amylose maize (Amylomaize) starch granules by human colonic bacteria. Appl Environ Microbiol. 1999 Nov;65(11):4848-54.

[58] Wang X, Conway PL, Brown IL, Evans AJ. In vitro utilization of amylopectin and high-amylose maize (Amylomaize) starch granules by human colonic bacteria. Appl Environ Microbiol. 1999 Nov;65(11):4848-54.

[59] Pimentel M, Constantino T, Kong Y, Bajwa M, Rezaei A, Park S. A 14-day elemental diet is highly effective in normalizing the lactulose breath test. Dig Dis Sci. 2004 Jan;49(1):73-7. Yancy WS Jr, Provenzale D, Westman EC. Improvement of gastroesophageal reflux disease after initiation of a low-carbohydrate diet: five brief cased reports. Altern Ther health med. 2001. Nov-Dec; 7(6):120,116-119. Austin GL, Thiny MT, Westman EC, Yancy WS Jr, Shaheen NJ. A very low-carbohydrate diet improves gastroesophageal reflux and its symptoms. Dig Dis Sci. 2006 Aug;51(8):1307-12.

[60] Fridge JL, Conrad C, Gerson L, Castillo RO, Cox K. Risk factors for small bowel bacterial overgrowth in cystic fibrosis. J Pediatr Gastroenterol Nutr. 2007 Feb;44(2):212-8.

[61] Goddard MS, Young G, Marcus R. The effect of amylose content on insulin and glucose responses to ingested rice. Am J Clin Nutr. 1984 Mar;39(3):388-92.

[62] Born P. Carbohydrate malabsorption in patients with non-specific abdominal complaints. World J Gastroenterol. 2007 Nov 21;13(43):5687-91. Chang FY, Lu CL. Irritable bowel syndrome in the 21st century: perspectives from Asia or South-east Asia. J Gastroenterol Hepatol. 2007 Jan;22(1):4-12.

[63] Badiali D, Corazziari E, Habib FI, Tomei E, Bausano G, Magrini P, Anzini F, Torsoli A. Effect of wheat bran in treatment of chronic nonorganic constipation. A double-blind controlled trial. Dig Dis Sci. 1995 Feb;40(2):349-56.

[64] Van Horn LV, Liu K, Parker D, Emidy L, Liao YL, Pan WH, Giumetti D, Hewitt J, Stamler J. Serum lipid response to oat product intake with a fat-modified diet. J Am Diet Assoc. 1986 Jun;86(6):759-64.

[65] (Leadbetter J, Ball MJ, Mann JI. Effects of increasing quantities of oat bran in hypercholesterolemic people. Am J Clin Nutr. 1991 Nov;54(5):841-5.

[66] Swain JF, Rouse IL, Curley CB, Sacks FM. Comparison of the effects of oat bran and low-fiber wheat on serum lipoprotein levels and blood pressure. N Engl J Med. 1990 Jan 18;322(3):147-52.

[67] Pietinen P, Rimm EB, Korhonen P, Hartman AM, Willett WC, Albanes D, Virtamo J. Intake of dietary fiber and risk of coronary heart disease in a cohort of Finnish men. The Alpha-Tocopherol, Beta-Carotene Cancer Prevention Study. Circulation. 1996 Dec 1;94(11):2720-7. Eshak ES, Iso H, Date C, Kikuchi S, Watanabe Y, Wada Y, Wakai K, Tamakoshi A; JACC Study Group. Dietary fiber intake is associated with reduced risk of mortality from cardiovascular disease among Japanese men and women. J Nutr. 2010 Aug;140(8):1445-53.

[68] Walker AR. Colon cancer and diet, with special reference to intakes of fat and fiber. Am J Clin Nutr. 1976 Dec;29(12):1417-26. Burkitt DP, Trowell HC. Dietary fibre and Western diseases. Ir Med J. 1977:70-272.

[69] Fuchs CS, Giovannucci EL, Colditz GA, Hunter DJ, Stampfer MJ, Rosner B, Speizer FE, Willett WC. Dietary fiber and the risk of colorectal cancer and adenoma in women. N Engl J Med. 1999 Jan 21;340(3):169-76.

[70] Uchida K, Kono S, Yin G, Toyomura K, Nagano J, Mizoue T, Mibu R, Tanaka M, Kakeji Y, Maehara Y, Okamura T, Ikejiri K, Futami K, Maekawa T, Yasunami Y, Takenaka K, Ichimiya H, Terasaka R. Dietary fiber, source

foods and colorectal cancer risk: the Fukuoka Colorectal Cancer Study. Scand J Gastroenterol. 2010 Oct;45(10):1223-31.

[71] Giovannucci E, Rimm EB, Stampfer MJ, Colditz GA, Ascherio A, Willett WC. Intake of fat, meat, and fiber in relation to risk of colon cancer in men. Cancer Res. 1994 May 1;54(9):2390-7.

[72] Shepherd SJ, Parker FC, Muir JG, Gibson PR. Dietary triggers of abdominal symptoms in patients with irritable bowel syndrome: randomized placebo-controlled evidence. Clin Gastroenterol Hepatol. 2008 Jul;6(7):765-71.

[73] Sayar S, Jannink JL, White PJ. Digestion residues of typical and high-beta-glucan oat flours provide substrates for in vitro fermentation. J Agric Food Chem. 2007 Jun 27;55(13):5306-11.

[74] Michel C, Kravtchenko TP, David A, et. al. In vitro prebiotic effects of Acacia gums onto the human intestinal microbiota depends on both botanical origin and environmental pH. 1998 Dec;4(6):257-66.

[75] Holloway WD, Tasman-Jones C, Lee SP. Digestion of certain fractions of dietary fiber in humans. Am J Clin Nutr. 1978 Jun;31(6):927-30.

[76] Soltoft J, Krag B, Gudmand-Hoyer E, Kristensen E, Wulff HR. A double-blind trial of the effect of wheat bran on symptoms of irritable bowel syndrome. Lancet. 1976 Feb 7;1(7954):270-2.

[77] Bijkerk CJ, de Wit NJ, Muris JW, Whorwell PJ, Knottnerus JA, Hoes AW. Soluble or insoluble fibre in irritable bowel syndrome in primary care? Randomised placebo controlled trial. BMJ. 2009 Aug 27;339:b3154.

[78] Dear KL, Elia M, Hunter JO. Do interventions which reduce colonic bacterial fermentation improve symptoms of irritable bowel syndrome? Dig Dis Sci. 2005 Apr;50(4):758-66.

[79] Hyams JS. Sorbitol intolerance: an unappreciated cause of functional gastrointestinal complaints. Gastroenterology. 1983 Jan;84(1):30-3.

[80] Born P, Zech J, Stark M, Classen M, Lorenz R. Carbohydrate substitutes: comparative study of intestinal absorption of fructose, sorbitol and xylitol. Med Klin (Munich). 1994 Nov 15;89(11):575-8.

[81] Yancy WS Jr, Provenzale D, Westman EC. Improvement of gastroesophageal reflux disease after initiation of a low-carbohydrate diet: five brief cased reports. Altern Ther health med. 2001. Nov-Dec; 7(6):120,116-119. Austin GL, Thiny MT, Westman EC, Yancy WS Jr,

Shaheen NJ. A very low-carbohydrate diet improves gastroesophageal reflux and its symptoms. Dig Dis Sci. 2006 Aug;51(8):1307-12. Austin GL, Dalton CB, Hu Y, Morris CB, Hankins J, Weinland SR, Westman EC, Yancy WS Jr, Drossman DA. A very low-carbohydrate diet improves symptoms and quality of life in diarrhea-predominant irritable bowel syndrome. Clin Gastroenterol Hepatol. 2009 Jun;7(6):706-708.

[82] Shepherd S, Gibson P. Fructose malabsorption and symptoms of irritable bowel syndrome: guidelines for effective dietary management. J Am Diet Assoc. 2006 Oct ;106 (10):1631-9.

[83] Gibson, P, Shepherd, S. Evidence-based dietary management of functional gastrointestinal symptoms: The FODMAP approach. J Gastroenterol Hepatol. 2010 Feb ;25 (2):252-8 20136989.

[84] Peter R Gibson, Susan J Shepherd. Evidence-based Dietary Management of Functional Gastrointestinal Symptoms: The FODMAP Approach. J Gastroenterol Hepatol. 2010;25(2):252-258.

[85] Gibson, P, Shepherd, S. Evidence-based dietary management of functional gastrointestinal symptoms: The FODMAP approach. J Gastroenterol Hepatol. 2010 Feb ;25 (2):252-8, 20136989f.

[86] Rada V, Bartonová J, Vlková E. Specific growth rate of bifidobacteria cultured on different sugars. Folia Microbiol (Praha). 2002;47(5):477-80.